Telling truth to power is nowhere more import maternity services. Lorin Lakasing reveals exactly what's wrong with the system and provides solutions that need to be heard.

    – Iain Dale, political journalist and broadcaster

A valuable, informative and at points challenging exposition of the evolution of maternity services in the UK over the last 30 years. Brilliantly timed and essential reading for anyone interested in the problems of maternity care and their potential solutions.

    – Prof. Hilary Marland, emeritus professor of history, Warwick
      University, and author of *Dangerous Motherhood*

Carefully researched and scattered with anecdotal evidence from years of clinical practice, this book explores why there are such high levels of dissatisfaction in maternity services, and why outcomes are not improving. Cultural change is not easy, but if we are to prevent the next scandal, we need to listen to both users and staff like Lorin Lakasing, who have devoted their lives to NHS maternity services, so that we can have an open and honest debate about the improvements we need.

    – Elizabeth Gardiner, CEO of Protect

A fascinating, insightful and extremely important read. As a husband of a victim of postpartum psychosis-induced suicide, this book really resonated with me; the idea that new mums must in some way give in to societal pressures and conform to expectations from set agendas is setting many parents up to fail. But understanding it from both sides, and the expectations put on midwives on the front line, highlights the complexities involved on all sides. Lorin explains this very well.

    – Richard Baish, member of Action on Postpartum Psychosis

An essential read for politicians, practitioners and indeed anyone seeking to understand the reasons for failures in maternity services. Its rigorous analysis of problems is shaped by evidence from her 30 years of personal experience. As a practitioner myself, I recognise the truth of her arguments and laud her ambition for the wholesale reforms needed to make NHS maternity services fit for purpose.

    – Judith Robbins, senior midwife

Lorin Lakasing gives voice to what many did not know about maternity care – and to what many knew but lacked the courage to say. This book is a brutally honest account that confronts uncomfortable truths with clarity and conviction. It will make uneasy reading as it forces all parties to face up to the part they played in the erosion of the maternity services, but it also inspires hope by proposing realistic strategies grounded in practical clinical expertise.

– Dr Maddalena Miele, consultant perinatal psychiatrist

Utterly compelling and full of detail. This is an eye-opening, objective assessment of maternity services.

– Prof Dominic Regan, solicitor and authority on civil litigation

Why NHS maternity

DELIVERING

care is broken and how

THE TRUTH

we can fix it together

Lorin Lakasing

Delivering the Truth

ISBN 978-1-915483-92-8

eISBN 978-1-915483-93-5

Published in 2025 by Right Book Press

Manufactured by
Sue Richardson Associates Ltd.
Studio 6,
9, Marsh Street
Bristol
BS1 4AA

info@therightbookcompany.com

EU Safety Representative
eucomply OÜ
Parnu mnt 139b-14
11317 Tallinn
Estonia

hello@eucompliancepartner.com
+33 756 90241

Contents

Preface

I did my first delivery as an undergraduate medical student under the supervision of a senior midwife in 1989 and have not looked back since. While my career has been immensely rewarding on a personal level, I recognise that in recent decades NHS maternity services have been the focus of much criticism, with the media increasingly describing a service that all too often fails its users. Such reports can be biased or misleading and often only scratch the surface. I care deeply about the quality and safety of NHS maternity care, and I felt compelled to write this book in an attempt to describe the NHS maternity service from the inside and provide a more balanced view of a very complex situation.

I have devoted the past 30 years to women's healthcare. During my postgraduate training in obstetrics and gynaecology, I worked in both teaching and district general hospitals. I became a member of the Royal College of Obstetricians and Gynaecologists in 1997. As a research fellow I participated in writing grant applications and undertook laboratory-based research in the field of maternal medicine. This work focused on investigating how disruption in the immune system and placental dysfunction contributed to miscarriage, stillbirth and preterm birth, and I was awarded a Doctorate of Medicine in 2000. As a clinical lecturer I was actively involved in revising the undergraduate curriculum for training in obstetrics and gynaecology, later becoming increasingly involved in postgraduate teaching. I completed subspeciality training in maternal-fetal medicine and was appointed a consultant in obstetrics and fetal medicine in 2004. I was elected a fellow of the Royal College of Obstetricians and Gynaecologists in 2012.

Throughout my career as a consultant, I have been involved in writing local and national clinical guidelines and collating data for audits. I became involved in the transition from paper-based medical records to electronic patient records within my healthcare region in the mid-2010s and have always had a keen interest in how clinical data is captured and used. I have undertaken external reviews of troubled maternity departments and reported on many cases presented at clinical risk management panels. As an educational supervisor for the Royal College of Obstetrics and Gynaecology, I regularly meet with postgraduate trainees to assess their progress and offer assistance and advice at different stages of their careers. As an accredited appraiser, I have listened to both junior and senior colleagues describe the triumphs and frustrations of providing maternity care and heard first-hand accounts of their experiences of working within the service. I have been involved in assessing cases referred to the General Medical Council (GMC) and observed colleagues who have been through disciplinary proceedings.

Aside from my clinical and teaching commitments, I regularly accept instructions from solicitors to act as an expert witness for the civil court and have provided more than 100 reports on potential obstetric malpractice claims. I also review cases referred to coroners' courts. This work requires me to read witness statements from both maternity staff and service users and has allowed me to gain valuable insights into the workings of the maternity service throughout the length and breadth of the UK, despite my personal practice being based in London. I have been a member of the Academy of Expert Witnesses since 2018 and have undertaken training in mediation and alternative dispute resolution to support my medicolegal work. I frequently give lectures on obstetric litigation, maternity safety strategies and avoidance of harm.

At various points during my career, I have had the opportunity to work abroad in obstetrics, paediatrics and women's health education, including in Australia, Denmark, Singapore, South Africa and Sri Lanka and have therefore had the privilege of observing healthcare in affluent as well as developing countries. I have an interest in global economic healthcare policy and support several women's healthcare charities both nationally and internationally.

In this book, I focus mainly on what I consider to be the three main stakeholders in NHS maternity care – service providers, service organisers and service users. I believe that each of these three parties has, inadvertently, contributed to a situation in which problems have become increasingly difficult to address and the proposed solutions have had limited effect or – worse still – have allowed poor care to flourish. I use anecdotes based on true-life events encountered in my many years of practice to explain my reasoning, although minor alterations have been made in some cases to maintain patient and staff confidentiality. No doubt many will disagree with these assessments or object to my opinions. Some will concur but may not feel at liberty to say so publicly. However, if genuine and sustained improvements are to be made, and I believe they can, an uncompromisingly inquisitive spotlight must be shone into the deep, dark corners of the NHS maternity service.

A note on language

Throughout the book, I use the terms 'mother' and 'woman' to reflect the majority of maternity service users and how they identify themselves but fully accept that there are many ways in which people express their gender and identity. Similarly, I use the pronouns she/her for midwives without intending to exclude the contribution of male, trans or gender-nonconforming midwives to the service. At the end of the book, I have included a glossary of medical terms.

The views represented in the work are entirely my own and do not represent those of the organisations I work in or have worked in previously.

The state of NHS maternity care

Introduction

Over the past couple of decades, it has been hard to escape media coverage of the state of maternity care in the UK's National Health Service (NHS). The public are bombarded with stories of terrible care provided to mothers and their babies. Newspaper articles (Johnson 2006; Spencer 2018; Bagot & Patient 2020; Roberts et al 2022; PA News Agency 2024) and programmes on prime-time television (Macdonald 2022; Lawless 2022; *Panorama* 2022; Cole 2022) have featured mothers giving harrowing accounts of the tragic loss of their newborns or tales of bereaved fathers raising children who only know their mother from a photograph. Women's magazines have also voiced concerns (Summers 2021; Lally 2022). In 2024, the report by the All-Party Parliamentary Group on Birth Trauma laid bare the long-term physical and psychological damage caused by poor maternity care (Birth Trauma 2024), and the service has been described as 'a cause for national shame' (Barry 2024). These reports have rightly provoked public dismay, anger and outrage. How has it come to this? Why have the problems gone on for so long? How come the service has not been able to mitigate against these disasters? After all, maternity, like all NHS services, is subject to regular healthcare inspections and these are supposed to pick up early warning signs long before failings prompt formal investigations.

Reports, reviews and inquiries

Over the past 30 years, numerous maternity units have been investigated and the reports that followed have made for sombre reading. In 2003, a healthcare watchdog report cleared Ashford and St Peter's Hospitals NHS Foundation Trust of any blame for an excess of neonatal deaths in its maternity unit but noted poor staffing levels, poor relationships between obstetricians and midwives, and excessive use of locum staff (Hansard 2003). The first report to attract national attention was the Healthcare Commission (HCC) review of maternity care at London North West University Healthcare NHS Trust published in August 2006 (HCC Report 2006). This review was prompted by ten maternal deaths between 2002 and 2005. Investigators identified a range of failures, including inappropriate working culture, staff shortages, discontent with a recent merger and weak leadership. The Trust was placed in special measures and the results of an inspection in 2008 were more favourable despite further maternal deaths. However, in 2021 the deaths of eight more babies in a five-week period prompted another review within the Trust and the maternity service was rated as 'requires improvement' by the Care Quality Commission (CQC). Investigators noted significant concerns regarding unit culture, bullying of staff and inappropriate patient interactions.

In 2007, The King's Fund, an independent charitable organisation which works to improve provision of healthcare in England, reported on the safety of maternity services and recommended improvements in staffing levels, training, teamwork and communication, better data collection and audit, and effective methods of learning from mistakes (Smith & Dixon 2007). Eight years later, the findings of the first large-scale independent national inquiry into maternity services rocked the nation. This landmark review was prompted by several maternal and neonatal deaths between 2004 and 2013 at Furness General Hospital in Barrow. Investigations commenced in 2013, and the Morecambe Bay report was published in 2015 (Kirkup 2015). It described a 'dysfunctional service', extremely poor working relationships, staff who were 'deficient in skills and knowledge', a growing move among midwives to pursue normal birth 'at any cost' and repeated failures to investigate poor outcomes properly. These factors constituted 'a lethal mix' of 'failures at almost every level', which had contributed to or caused the loss of lives. Crucially, the report went on to state that these problems 'did not develop overnight'. The Trust was placed in special measures between 2014 and 2016 and although some improvements were noted soon afterwards, the CQC downgraded the service from 'good' to 'inadequate' at subsequent inspections.

In January 2019, the Royal College of Midwives (RCM) and the Royal College of Obstetricians and Gynaecologists (RCOG) jointly commissioned a review of maternity services at the Royal Glamorgan Hospital and Prince Charles Hospital run by Cwm Taf Morgannwg University Health Board in Wales (RCM/RCOG 2019). The initial investigation followed concerns about 21 stillbirths, five neonatal deaths and 17 serious maternal complications in labour but was extended to include care provided to a further 27 women, most of whom were admitted to the intensive care unit. These cases occurred from 2016 to 2018 and the investigations revealed all-too-familiar findings – distrust and disengagement of staff in relation to an imminent merger, lack of availability of senior obstetricians even within working hours, 'poor knowledge of or lack of adherence to clinical guidelines', 'high rates of locum cover', 'lack of a functioning governance system', unskilled neonatal care, inadequate midwifery staffing and a culture within the service which was 'perceived as punitive'. The Trust was placed in special measures and an independent panel was set up by the Welsh government to oversee improvements.

In 2020, following concerns raised by four whistleblowers, the CQC made an unannounced visit to Worcestershire Royal Hospital maternity unit and inspectors noted inadequate staffing, patchy reporting of clinical incidents, poor data keeping, a service that 'did not have an open culture where staff felt they could raise concerns without fear' and leaders that 'did not engage with staff effectively' (CQC 2021a). That same year a coroner ruled that the death of a one-week-old infant was due to negligent care provided by maternity staff at the East Kent Hospitals University NHS Foundation Trust, a unit already known to be underperforming (CQC 2021b). The CQC inspection concluded that staff shortages, lack of senior obstetrician involvement and failure to complete mandatory training compromised care. In 2021, the CQC report on maternity services at Newham University Hospital highlighted poor leadership, a 'culture of blame', 'safety champions not visible' and 'difficulties in communication', especially with non-English-speaking service users (CQC 2021c).

Just when it seemed things could get no worse, March 2022 brought the publication of the final report on poor maternity outcomes at Shrewsbury and Telford Hospital NHS Trust (Ockenden 2022). There had been an interim report on the care of 250 mothers in December 2020 (Ockenden 2020), but the sheer scale of the problems unearthed warranted an extended investigation. The final report was based on the assessment of care provided to 1,862 former patients over a 20-year period and included stillbirths, neonatal deaths, maternal deaths and other serious complications. It described a dismal service – staff 'lacking in compassion and kindness', 'deflecting blame onto families', locums filling rota gaps, 'anaesthetists invited at the last minute', 'failure to work collaboratively across disciplines', a culture of 'them and us' between midwives and obstetricians, inadequate staffing and training, incident reporting that was 'cursory' with 'some significant cases not investigated at all', maternity governance teams that 'inappropriately downgraded serious incidents in order to avoid external scrutiny', failure to conduct fetal heart rate monitoring in labour, use of high-dose oxytocin despite abnormal fetal heart rate readings, a 'service-wide failure to follow appropriate procedures and guidelines', 'repeated failures to escalate concerns both in the antenatal and postnatal period', a 'leadership team up to board level in a constant state of churn and change' and a lack of strategic direction when planning the maternity service. What was truly remarkable about this report, however, was not these findings, because, depressingly, previous investigations had raised exactly the same issues. No, the truly remarkable thing was that the maternity services at the Trust had been subject to several other inspections during the period under investigation and the findings were rather different. Following unfavourable reports in the local press and two litigation cases in 2004, the HCC visited the unit in 2007 and declared the standards of care satisfactory and that the unit did not meet the criteria for a full investigation (HCC 2007).

In 2013, two clinical commissioning groups reviewed the Trust's risk management processes and concluded there was 'a robust approach to risk management, clinical governance and learning from incidents' and that the higher-than-expected admission to the neonatal intensive care unit was a result of 'diligent reporting' (Maternity Services Review, the Shrewsbury and Telford Hospital NHS Trust 2013). In 2014, the NHS Litigation Authority (NHS LA) awarded the Trust a Level 3 clinical risk management standard, the highest achievable (NHS LA 2014). This was based on data for implementation of guidelines, audit and clinical outcomes submitted largely via self-reporting systems. In 2015, the CQC awarded the Trust a 'good' rating (CQC 2015), but two years later the RCOG review of 2017 concluded that there were workforce issues, inadequate incident reporting, inadequate risk management and governance systems, very low morale and perinatal mortality rates that remained persistently above average (RCOG 2017). This last set of findings was initially rejected by the Trust board and actions were taken to attach a more favourable addendum to the report before final submission. In 2018, the CQC downgraded the unit to 'inadequate' due to lack of evidence of learning from serious incidents, problems with unit culture, difficulties in relation to a maternity service operating across split sites and a general lack of accountability (CQC 2018). Why the conflicting reports?

And there's more. In September 2020, Nottingham Maternity Hospitals received a CQC rating of 'inadequate' based on poor staffing, bad record keeping, delays in care and treatment, leaders who 'did not always effectively identify and mitigate risks' and deliberate underreporting of stillbirths (CQC 2022). This sparked another national maternity inquiry, which is currently under way and looks set to include more than 2,500 cases (Sissons & Ashe 2025). The sheer scale is likely to dwarf previous investigations. And most recently at the time of writing, Leeds Teaching Hospital NHS Trust has had its maternity and neonatal services downgraded due to a series of poor outcomes and a signficant number of 'red flags' in relation to staffing (CQC 2025).

There are around 150 maternity units in the UK and a recent CQC inspection of 131 units in England rated almost half as 'requires improvement' (36 per cent) or 'inadequate' (12 per cent) (CQC 2024). These long-standing concerns have prompted the Maternity Safety Alliance, a group made up of bereaved families and their supporters, to call for a statutory public inquiry into maternity safety in England (maternitysafetyalliance.co.uk). In June 2025, following a series of meetings with service users who have experienced poor clinical outcomes, the health and social care secretary announced a rapid national investigation into NHS and maternity and neonatal services which would go part way to addressing this. The investigation was set to look at the worst-performing units in the country and then outline a national set of actions to improve care across the sector (NHS England 2025).

What is really going on?

There are those who question or try to sugar-coat the findings of investigations into maternity care, but the first step towards solving problems is acknowledging they exist… everywhere. Thanks to these inquiries, it is clear *what* the problems are but not *why* they have come about and *how* to tackle them. In this book, I hope to address the following questions:

+ How have UK maternity outcomes changed over time, and how does NHS maternity data compare with other countries?
+ Why is understaffing such a concern and why are staff lacking in skills and knowledge?
+ Why is the service so reliant on bank/agency/locum staff?
+ Why are teamwork and staff morale so poor?
+ Why do staff find mergers and relocations so destabilising?
+ Why is senior input often inadequate? Where are the senior clinicians and what are they doing instead?
+ Why is there so much bullying? Who are the perpetrators? Why does it continue?
+ What do 'unit culture' and 'blame culture' mean?
+ Why are there persistent accounts of disrespectful interactions between staff and service users?
+ Why the obsession with 'natural birth', and what choice do mothers really have?
+ Why does fetal heart rate monitoring pose such problems?
+ How and why are serious incidents downgraded, misrepresented or under-reported?
+ How can a maternity unit that healthcare inspectors rate as 'good' then find itself subject to a national inquiry? If the findings are so contradictory, are inspections of any value at all?

+ Why is there a lack of leadership or strategic vision in so many maternity units?
+ Why has maternity care not improved despite implementation of recommendations from independent inquiries?

Conclusion

The cost of poor maternity care is immeasurable. It affects lives and livelihoods, it shatters hopes and dreams, it destroys families and puts pressure on their relationship with wider society. Mortality is a heartbreaking outcome and often makes the headlines, but it is long-term morbidity that impacts on quality of life, and physical and psychological wellbeing. Poor outcomes also affect staff who are left helpless, fearful and insecure. There are no winners when the maternity service is broken.

I believe we are now at a tipping point where what we do next determines whether there is an NHS maternity service to speak of in years to come. Interestingly, although it may be hard to believe, this small but significant medical speciality has led the way in healthcare development in the past, as I will discuss in later chapters. Where maternity goes, other specialities follow, so there is an imperative to getting this right for the wider NHS too. Before looking at each of the major stakeholders – service providers, service organisers and service users – and the role they have played in creating the current state of affairs, I will first describe the historical background to maternity care in the UK and the evolution into the modern-day NHS maternity service.

Background to the modern-day maternity service

Introduction

There is no country or culture in which the arrival of a baby is not regarded as an important and special event, but pregnancy and childbirth can be complicated. Data from the World Health Organization (WHO) shows pregnancy-related problems remain the leading cause of death globally in young women aged 15–19 years (WHO 2024), with 95 per cent of deaths occurring in some of the poorest countries in the world. The differences between the lowest and highest ranked countries are staggering: around one in ten mothers in sub-Saharan Africa and three in 100,000 mothers in Scandinavia (WHO 2025). But maternity care is evolving the world over and this notion of maternity outcomes being on a trajectory of improvement is beautifully described by the extraordinary Swedish public health physician and academic Hans Rosling in his posthumously published book *Factfulness* (Rosling & Rønnlund 2018). Here he notes similarities between healthcare in Sweden in the late 1940s (at the time of his birth) with that of Egypt in the 2000s (when he wrote the book) and explains, in his characteristically witty and insightful way, that he was 'born in Egypt'. Understanding this is crucial because assessing maternity outcomes must be placed in context. It would be wrong to congratulate ourselves just because things are worse elsewhere or were worse in the past. Many reports describing maternity care cheerfully note that, overall, the NHS is a safe healthcare system in which to have a baby. This is odd for two reasons. First, UK maternity data in recent years has not shown sustained improvements and, second, pregnancy and childbirth are physiological rather than pathological processes, so outcomes should be quite good anyway. Indeed, the optimist might conclude that even in sub-Saharan Africa, where little or no care is provided, 90 per cent of mothers survive. But for a country with a well-developed publicly funded health service, 'all right in most cases' is not necessarily good enough.

Historical data

Uniquely among medical specialities, maternity demographic data has been collected in the UK since the mid-1800s and, although it is inevitably imperfect, it gives us a handle on general trends (statista. com). For much of the 19th century, the number of liveborn infants was just over one million per year, but this has shown steady decline to 594,677 livebirths in England and Wales in 2024 (ONS 2025a). In the 1800s, the average British woman of childbearing age would have had 5.5 babies; by the early 1900s this was an average of three, and since the 1980s this has remained below two. Average maternal age at first birth has risen from early twenties in the 1800s to 25 years in the 1940s and 33.8 years in 2023. The changes reflect rising standards of living, better education for women and improved access to contraception.

The worst outcome in any pregnancy is maternal death. Historical reports into maternal death in England make for grim reading (Loudon 1986). Reports from the 1700s range from 25–50/1,000 births, the wide variation reflecting that many pregnancies and births went unreported. This desperate situation continued well into the next century and, in 1857, epidemiologist William Farr described 'a deep, dark and continuous stream of mortality' in his report to the Registrar General (Farr 1857). Most maternal deaths occurred due to sepsis or haemorrhage, but things were about to change. The introduction of sulphur-based antibiotics in the early 1900s resulted in a dramatic fall in maternal deaths to 5–30/1,000 births by 1935. The practice of administering ergot extract from tea, which acts as a uterotonic to stem postpartum haemorrhage, was another game changer. The maternal death rate continued to fall, necessitating a welcome change in the denominator to 10,000, and then 100,000. By 2003–2005, the UK maternal death rate had fallen to 13.95/100,000 and in 2017–2019, it was at its lowest at 8.79/100,000, although recent data shows a rise to 12.67/100,000 in 2021–2023 (MBRRACE-UK 2025).

Although these figures do not necessarily tell us much about the quality of maternity care per se, infant mortality rates in England have also been recorded since the 1800s, and these have fallen from a shocking 329/1,000 births, ie one in three babies, when records first began, to 162/1,000 in 1915, then 65/1,000 in 1945 and 3.9/1,000 in 2022 (ONS 2025b). A more useful indicator of maternity care might be the stillbirth rate, and national data has been collected since 1927 when the rate was around 40/1,000. This has fallen to around 4/1,000 in the 1990s but has struggled to fall further for sustained periods of time (ONS 2025a). In Scandinavia it is around 2/1,000.

Let us consider more closely what this data does and doesn't tell us. The first thing to notice is that the greatest improvements pre-date the establishment of the NHS in 1948 and thus it is very likely that societal changes, such as improvements in housing, better nutrition, provision of clean water, improved hygiene and women's education, played a more substantial role than universal access to healthcare. Second, the game changers in relation to maternal mortality were therapeutic interventions, notably antibiotics and uterotonics, showing that, while pregnancy is a physiological process, it is foolish to assume the body will get it right every time without assistance. Third, mortality is a binary outcome, but there is no historical data on the considerable morbidity associated with pregnancy and childbirth. These are softer outcomes often associated with a broader spectrum of longer-term disorders, such as perinatal mental health disease, urinary incontinence or vaginal wall prolapse for the mother, or disability for the infant.

Finally, international comparative data are not reassuring. The World's Mothers Report by the Save the Children charity published in 2013 ranked the UK 23rd, with similar outcomes to Greece and the Balkan states (Save the Children 2013). WHO data post-2018 confirms that several countries, including New Zealand, Norway, the

Netherlands, Germany, Sweden, Switzerland and Austria, had lower maternal death rates. The Organisation for Economic Co-operation and Development (OECD), which uses maternal and infant mortality as key economic indicators, ranked UK maternity services poorly (OECD 2023). While any improvements are to be welcomed, clearly there is no room for complacency.

The origins of midwifery and obstetrics in the UK

To better explain the maternity service as it stands today, I will briefly summarise the evolution of the two interconnected professions of midwifery and obstetrics.

A potted history of midwifery in the UK

The practice of midwifery is as old as the human race itself, and there are wonderful accounts of the work of this elite profession from ancient Egypt, Greece and the Roman Empire. The word 'mid-wife' is likely to be either German or Anglo-Saxon in origin meaning 'with wife'. Midwives were known to have attended upon the births of the wives of the medieval kings of England, and the first midwifery manual written in English was printed in 1540, a translation via Latin of a German work. By the 1600s, it was not unusual for city-dwelling women of a certain social status to pay for the services of a midwife during labour, although working-class women especially in rural areas went through birth either alone or with an unskilled attendant.

By the mid-1700s, the 'man midwife', a new breed of midwifery practitioner seemingly in possession of extra skills, emerged. Not surprisingly, many traditional midwives felt threatened by them and the interventions they introduced. This clash of ideologies, namely letting nature take its course versus assisting and intervening with the process of birthing, remains an enduring conflict. In the writing that accompanied a picture from the early 18th century depicting William Hunter, the famous Scottish anatomist and physician, attending a birth, the author describes how it was 'not until a strenuous fight with the midwives was it customary for a man-midwife to be present at a confinement'. Nevertheless, male birth attendants remained undeterred and continued to foster an academic interest in the process of birthing, documenting for the first time how it went wrong and what could be done to fix it. Soon midwifery was being taught as a specialist branch of surgery, and because women were not allowed access to higher education this widened the gap between professional men and their educationally disadvantaged female counterparts. Traditional midwifery was further undermined by unflattering social narratives of the time such as the portrayal of Sairey Gamp in the novel *Martin Chuzzlewit* by Charles Dickens published between 1843 and 1844, in which she was depicted as a drunk, sloppy, incompetent nurse-cum-midwife, someone intellectually inferior whose practice was outdated and unscientific. To counter this, the Matron's Aid Society or the Trained Midwives' Registration Society, later the Midwives' Institute, was established in 1881. This organisation aimed to improve teaching, training and the status of midwives, and the profession survived not least of all because midwives continued to support women from all social backgrounds.

The profession gained legal recognition in the UK in 1902 with the first Midwives Act. Further Acts followed in 1918, 1926 and 1936. During World War One, despite thousands of nurses being deployed to field hospitals throughout the country and abroad, midwives were 'protected' and encouraged to stay in their local towns and cities to get on with the difficult work of community midwifery and conducting deliveries at home, where more than 90 per cent of births took place. Interestingly, the opposite occurred during World War Two, when many pregnant women were evacuated from big towns and cities for their own protection against bombardment. They were transferred to stand-alone maternity units built in the countryside by the government and staffed by midwives brought in to provide care. After World War Two, the Midwives' Institute was granted a royal charter and became the Royal College of Midwives in 1947.

Following the establishment of the NHS in 1948, many rural maternity units remained active but shortages in midwifery staffing became increasingly problematic. Thousands of nurses from abroad were invited to fill the gaps, but only the crème de la crème specialised in midwifery. Caribbean and Irish nurses were favoured due to their notably robust background in general nursing. By the late 1950s–early

1960s, a time depicted in the TV series *Call the Midwife*, less than 30 per cent of births were conducted at home. The UK homebirth rate today is less than 2.5 per cent.

While understandably falling under the umbrella of general nursing, UK midwives have fought long and hard to maintain their own identity and autonomy as practitioners with a very distinct skill set. Unlike in many other countries, they have remained unquestionably the backbone of the NHS maternity service.

A potted history of obstetrics in the UK

The history of obstetrics in the UK dates back to the 1600s with the introduction of the aforementioned 'man-midwife'. By the early 1700s, there were descriptions of these practitioners fashioning surgical instruments to assist in complex deliveries – sharp blades to perform craniotomies for hydrocephalus, forceps for obstructed labour and hooks for breech extraction. At first, many regarded these man-midwives or accoucheurs as controversial, comical, fashionable or even subversive characters whose role was superfluous to requirement. They often assumed the title of surgeon while working covertly in women's bedchambers only when summoned by 'proper' midwives to attend emergencies. But by the end of the 18th century, acceptance of this new profession grew, especially among the aristocracy, who regarded the co-attendance during labour of a qualified professional as desirable. These practitioners were paid many times more than their female co-workers; they moved in influential circles and established social connections which furthered their cause.

Soon there were formal training programmes focused on anatomy and surgery, and the term 'obstetrics', derived from Latin and meaning 'one who stands opposite', appeared in the medical literature. By the middle of the 19th century, obstetric teaching was a compulsory part of the medical student curriculum. Practitioners collected and analysed maternity outcome data, and it became clear that pregnancy and childbirth were complex processes that warranted attention not just during labour. At the beginning of the 20th century, visionary maternity units in Scotland set up 'antenatal clinics', primarily to detect pre-eclampsia, a major contributor to maternal death. This potentially fatal condition was perfectly portrayed in the TV series

Downton Abbey when Sybil, the youngest of the three sisters and herself a qualified nurse, died shortly after childbirth from 'toxaemia of pregnancy'. Obstetrics continued to be regarded as a branch of surgery until 1929 when the British College of Obstetrics and Gynaecology was founded. The organisation was granted a royal charter in 1947 and thus the RCOG was established. This organisation has been at the forefront of teaching, training, assessment and continuing professional education for practitioners ever since.

In the NHS, the role of the obstetrician is to support midwives and take over conduct of a case when there is deviation from the physiological norm. This makes obstetrics different from any other medical speciality insofar as the primary carer is from a nursing background, with the medical practitioner in a secondary role. Appreciating this difference is crucial to understanding many of the issues that have arisen in NHS maternity care today.

The modern-day NHS maternity service

The approximate budget for NHS maternity is around £3 billion per annum, which is less than 2 per cent of the overall NHS budget of around £200 billion per annum, but despite its diminutive size, it is the highest stakes speciality of all because of the young lives involved.

Certain words or phrases are commonly used to describe public services. For example, women talk about their maternity unit being 'outstanding' or 'poor' or 'inadequate', or 'in need of improvement'. These phrases may influence where women choose to deliver because they believe the service is better in one maternity unit than another. Reporters often interview NHS representatives who extol the virtues of 'the Service' or respond to criticisms or deficiencies in it. And politicians endlessly talk about reforms or improvements to 'the Service'. But what exactly does 'the Service' mean? What or who makes up 'the Service'? Does it all need improving? Do some parts work better than others? What can be done about the parts that don't work? Are all the various parts necessary? Are some key parts missing? How is it possible to ensure 'the Service' remains fit for purpose now and in the future? When was the last time you heard such issues debated? No one in the media seems able or willing to distil 'the Service' down to its various components, preferring instead to report on it as if it were some vastly complex heterogeneous mass unable to be disentangled. But this is not the case. Most NHS services, including maternity, can be deconstructed into three basic components:

1. **People**
2. **Tools**
3. **Spaces**

Put simply, you need staff with the correct skills to have easy access to the right tools so they can attend to patients in a space that is designed to allow care to be delivered safely and effectively.

People

This means staff. Individuals who either directly or indirectly receive their salaries from the NHS via funding from the Department of Health and Social Care (DHSC) courtesy of the UK taxpayer. 'People' can be further subdivided into:

a) Frontline staff

These are professionals who have *direct* contact with patients, ie 'service providers' – midwives, obstetricians, anaesthetists, neonatologists, pharmacists, sonographers, physiotherapists, porters, cleaners, administrative staff, canteen staff, phlebotomists, laundry staff and so on. Individuals who are quite literally 'seen' by the service users. Chapter 3 is devoted to frontline staff.

b) Managers

These individuals are *indirectly* responsible for patient care, ie 'service organisers'. Their job is to ensure frontline staff work effectively and productively with access to the correct tools in fit-for-purpose workspaces that facilitate safe care. Chapter 4 is devoted to managers.

Tools

Compared with other medical specialities, the maternity service does not require many tools. However, care provision is contingent upon a steady supply of pharmaceutical agents, notably drugs for pain relief and induction of labour, and uterotonics. Infection is treated with old-fashioned and thus cheaper antibiotics because these are tried and tested in terms of fetal teratogenicity. Far less electronic and technical equipment is used compared with many surgical specialities, although as ultrasound technology evolves, upgrading of equipment remains an ongoing cost. Fetal monitoring equipment requires modest investment. A standard caesarean surgical operating tray has not changed for more than 50 years, and although disposable ventouse suction cups for operative vaginal delivery are favoured now, the standard obstetric forceps has barely altered in design for centuries, as the series of similar instruments found under the floorboards in the attic of the Chamberlen family in 1831 testifies. Other consumables include bedlinen, gowns, gloves, the fabled 'warm towels', which feature in all films in which a baby is born, needles and syringes, dressings, mops for cleaners, and plates and cups for canteen services, all of which are mundane but essential. But in short, maternity is not a profligate speciality.

Spaces

Poor NHS infrastructure is a major problem rarely highlighted in the media because it is considerably less attention grabbing than maternal or neonatal deaths, staff shortages or strike action. In 2023/2024 the NHS spent £13.8 billion on estates maintenance (Fozzard et al 2024), and maternity units are not exempt from decay. Anyone who has pushed a labouring woman on a three-wheeled trolley past crumbling plasterboard on the way to an operating theatre where the door is held open by a wedge fashioned from an old surgical clog, or sutured an episiotomy with the help of an iPhone light held in place by a medical student, will know exactly what I am talking about. So bad is the state of many clinical areas that this is often a key factor in forcing unit closures, mergers and relocations. This infrastructure problem falls under the direct control of either local or central government, often a combination, and the situation nationally is dismal (Barron 2022). But it is not just bricks and mortar: fixtures and fittings, such as ramps for wheelchair access, waiting room chairs, examination benches, shelves, medical lamps, trolleys, washbasins, disposal sinks, incinerators, laundry carts, reception desks and patient information display screens, are also affected. While this is undoubtedly a huge issue, I have chosen in this book to focus on the other elements of 'the Service' because, if there is one stark take-home message post the Covid-19 pandemic, it is that there is little point having shiny, new, purpose-built hospitals such as the Nightingale units unless you have enough frontline staff to run them.

Conclusion

While UK maternity outcome data has demonstrated improvements, there is still some way to go to achieve the standards of comparable nations. In outlining the historical background to midwifery and obstetrics here, my aim has been to explain some of the interprofessional differences I discuss in later chapters. Most importantly, I hope that distilling 'the Service' into its component parts has identified two of the three major stakeholders in the modern-day service. In the next chapter, I will discuss the first of these, frontline staff, who are the service providers.

3 Service providers – caregiving on the frontline

Introduction

A notable theme raised in all independent national maternity inquiries and workforce planning reports is the enduring challenge of adequate staffing. Chronic problems have been identified in serial workforce reports by both the RCM and RCOG. Reports concentrate on absolute numbers or, more usefully, 'level of skill' or 'skill mix'. Acquiring skills means being trained to do the job, and the job itself needs to be attractive enough for people to want to do it and to continue doing it long term. In this chapter, I discuss how these aspects of the profession have changed over the years to get us to where we are today.

Frontline midwifery

Training

A prerequisite for entry into midwifery training some 30–40 years ago was the completion of three years of general nursing training, resulting in a diploma in nursing. Only the very best applied for a further three years of training in midwifery, which were onerous and definitely not for the faint hearted. The hours were unpredictable, the work fraught with uncertainty and drama: student midwives had to prove themselves worthy of being members of the most exclusive field of nursing. After qualifying, there were a further 18 months working under the supervision of a named mentor. These were experienced professionals, role models responsible for signing off clinical skills. They led by example, supporting student midwives in their everyday practice. Older midwives often describe them as a constant presence watching over their shoulders.

Thus, only after seven and a half years of training would midwives take on sole charge of a pregnant woman. To ensure ongoing support, many maternity units organised their midwives into teams, with members having a range of skills or years in practice. Over time, most were encouraged to gain extra proficiencies in antenatal screening or lactation support, or develop special interests in community midwifery or bereavement care. After many years of frontline work, they might become lead for antenatal education for mothers-to-be, teach neonatal first aid, train more junior staff, perhaps even become a mentor themselves. The competence their vocational apprenticeship and subsequent practice had bestowed upon them translated into confidence as an independent practitioner, and now it was their job to help those following in their footsteps. This generation of senior midwives often had a fearsome reputation, and I worked with many as a junior doctor. Like Sister M, a woman of few words with piercing blue eyes who would look her junior midwives up and down at the start of each shift. Anyone wearing nail polish or jewellery was sent home and told to 'come back when ready to work'. Or Sister F, who would not let us step onto 'her' postnatal ward until we had said 'good morning' to the receptionist, the canteen lady and the cleaner. These people were far more important than us because they were permanent members of 'her' team. Junior doctors came and went on rotation; they did not matter. She enforced visiting times strictly because, 'How on Earth are mothers supposed to look after their babies if they don't get enough rest?' Bedlinen was turned over twice a day. She timed how long it took the junior midwives to do this. Too long, and the mother might be making her way back from the shower with nowhere to rest. Too short, had they really folded the corners in properly? Visiting fathers and relatives did as they were told: it was not in anyone's interest to pick fights with Sister F. As far as these two formidable professionals were concerned, manners, discipline and understanding the hierarchy were central to good midwifery. Today they would be regarded as stuffy, inflexible bullies and their undermining behaviour would not be tolerated. Back then, it was the norm.

Midwifery, like nursing in general, has struggled to maintain its appeal as a career. Despite there being some way to go to achieve equality in the workplace, the opportunities open to young women today far exceed those of their forebears, with many alternative careers offering better working hours, flexibility, career progression, social status and remuneration. Other traditionally 'female' careers, such as childcare, catering or teaching, have suffered the same plight. These jobs are vital in maintaining our communities and the wider society in which our youngest members develop, but society no longer attaches as much value to them. Recruitment within the UK has been a major problem, resulting in a dependency on filling vacant positions in health and social care with workers from overseas. To address the nursing and midwifery shortfall, Project 2000 was introduced in 1986 (UK Central Council 1986), a higher education scheme which replaced the apprenticeship model of training with formal knowledge-based assessments. Instead of 'just' a diploma in nursing, successful students would be awarded a degree, which would enable them to apply for higher postgraduate training. After only 18 months of foundation training in general nursing, students could opt for specialist training in midwifery, thus bypassing the long years of training previously required. For the first time, a student could become a registered midwife, with a degree, in three years. Why bother learning about neuro-observations in patients with strokes or how to dress a leg ulcer in a person with diabetes? Surely these skills are superfluous to midwifery?

Despite much objection from senior midwifery teachers at the time, this new style of training was rolled out but, just as they predicted, it turned out that core general nursing knowledge is necessary after all. In the decades that have followed, virtually every national audit has highlighted the contribution of non-obstetric conditions to poor maternal outcomes. It turns out that understanding cardiac disease or knowing how to manage asthma, epilepsy and diabetes, all relatively common conditions in young women, is important. So is being able to perform neuro-observations in a mother following an eclamptic seizure or pass a nasogastric tube to relieve postoperative ileus following caesarean section. Not to mention early recognition of sepsis or management of acute haemorrhage. Today's training programmes have been reduced to a quick skim over these critical matters in the first 18 months, followed by a further 18 months in which the midwifery part of training focuses largely on normal physiological pregnancy and birth in healthy women. Emphasis is increasingly placed on provision of pregnancy care in a social context, with patient advocacy and supporting maternal choice at the core. While these changes in training are understandable, the net result is a generation of midwives whose clinical comfort zone is limited and whose mindset is so ideologically committed to normal pregnancy and birth that they are less able to recognise and deal with clinical deviations from the norm, until the clinical picture becomes overtly pathological. I recall an experienced midwife educator saying, 'If you assessed these students according to the criteria by which I was assessed, not one of them would pass, but according to their marking system, I would surely fail.'

The job

The pressures of work as a frontline midwife today are colossal. The workload is erratic and physically demanding, requiring continuous multitasking. The role is also seemingly limitless. Alongside the obvious job of caring for mother and baby, there is patient advocacy, emotional and psychological support, standing in for absent members of staff, supervising less experienced staff, acting as confidante, teaching and training, and safeguarding. On a busy shift, moving patients to and from wards and helping to clean rooms or make beds between deliveries are commonplace. There is an endless amount of digital 'paperwork': the requirement to document everything, fill in pro formas and checklists, and complete a series of repetitive administrative tasks which divert attention away from clinical care. It can take up to 30 minutes to discharge a mother and baby from the postnatal ward. Most midwives spend far longer staring at computer screens than interacting with mothers and babies, and many report anxiety and stress because they feel these aspects have overshadowed their 'real job' (The UK WHELM Study 2018).

As a result, morale is affected and some switch to survival

mode or do the bare minimum. Disengagement is a major problem. Relationships between staff members can become strained, with some feeling put upon while others shirk their duties. Tempers are frayed, resulting in incivility (Newitt et al 2024). It makes for horrid reading when independent national maternity inquiries report frontline staff being rude or dismissive to mothers. This is unforgivable, but the other side of the story is that frontline midwives are regularly subject to abuse from service users (RCM 2020). Pregnant women can be anxious, stubborn, angry, distressed or even violent. This may reflect frustration with the 'hit and miss' nature of maternity care but being at the receiving end is upsetting. NHS hospital corridors and waiting rooms are plastered with posters encouraging patients to be kind and considerate towards staff. Some state 'abuse of staff will not be tolerated' but these are unenforceable aspirations. The situation is made worse by the fact that, unlike most other specialities, frontline maternity staff deal with partners and relatives as much as they do with the mothers. In modern maternity care, mothers expect support from partners and relatives every step of the way, but these omnipresent others bring a new dimension to all interactions. Midwives who work in the community expose themselves to additional risks associated with entering people's homes, often visiting no-go areas. Maternity care is by its very nature a 24-hour speciality, yet there is no extra protection offered to frontline midwives, day or night.

The daily grind soon takes its toll. Sickness and absenteeism are common (NHS Digital 2025). Clinics are understaffed and never finish on time. Labour ward care is particularly challenging and interactions with obstetricians and other members of the team can be strained because acting as the primary advocate for a mother can put midwives in conflict with professionals from other disciplines who might be more intervention friendly or quicker to recommend a different course of action – a situation that national inquiries often refer to as the 'them and us' culture of caregiving. Midwives often describe being 'piggy in the middle' as different sets of priorities collide – for example, when a midwife might feel she wants to support a mother pushing in active second stage for a while longer but equally understands why the obstetrician has suggested trial of instrumental vaginal delivery in the operating theatre because the fetal heart rate pattern is concerning.

Those with enough stamina to progress in their careers may one day be tasked with the role of labour ward coordinator, the most unenviable and undervalued job in maternity care. This poor soul has the gargantuan responsibility of knowing exactly what is happening in every corner of the labour ward at all times. They oversee all acute admissions, deploy midwives appropriately, summon obstetric/anaesthetic/neonatal help when needed and manage all transfers to and from obstetric theatres. It is unquestionably the most crucial role in maintaining safety and, as an obstetric trainee, I learnt quickly that the first question one should ask when taking over the labour ward shift is 'Who is the labour ward coordinator?' I have witnessed some formidable individuals who make the job look almost easy and when in charge the avoidance of disasters is all but guaranteed, no matter how busy the shift. Sadly, the opposite is true of others who deflect as much responsibility as possible, preferring to spend time behind a computer screen or on their mobile phones. Unfortunately, the staffing crisis means the service sometimes has to make do with staff whose skills or dedication are not what they should be. But even the most able labour ward coordinator cannot magic up staff where they do not exist. The RCM estimates that the NHS in England is short of the equivalent of 2,500 full-time midwives (Bona 2023) so it is little wonder that staff surveys suggest 30–50 per cent of shifts are understaffed. As a result, labour ward coordinators often get sucked into direct care provision and this inevitably spells disaster because the 'helicopter view' of the unit is lost and the remaining frontline staff start working in siloes, unaware of other competing priorities at any moment in time. The consequences are often tragic: one simply needs to read the accounts from independent national inquiries for proof.

The need to plug gaps in the duty rotas means the service becomes over-reliant on bank or agency staff who are qualified to do the job on paper but in practice might have little operational knowledge of the unit. In an obstetric emergency, knowing the relevant extension number for the blood transfusion laboratory or numbers for the neonatal crash team off by heart can save critical minutes in response times. Even in the absence of such drama, these staff are often 'carried' by core staff as they may not know local protocols or have access to the software systems for recording clinical information. I recall one event when a mother experienced a drug reaction on a postnatal ward staffed by two agency midwives, neither of whom knew the code to the emergency drug cupboard or the shortcut to the operating theatres where the required antidote was kept. In short, any service that relies on non-core staff is inherently unsafe. In 2015, the RCM reported that almost £18 million was spent on agency staff, which could have paid for 511 experienced full-time midwives (RCM 2015).

Midwifery staff shortages have resulted in basic care being prioritised over and above extended roles, such as assisting at caesarean sections or specialising in high-dependency care, care for women with psychiatric problems or addictions, or teenage pregnancy. For those mothers who have suffered the ultimate loss, the need for specialist midwifery bereavement care is paramount. There are no cheers of joy or emotional utterances of hope for the future when a stillborn baby is delivered, just a depth of human grief no one can imagine until they find themselves in that most awful of situations. Bereavement midwives know how to be comfortable with silence, they find just the right words, and at the same time check blood pressure, pulse and blood loss. This is midwifery at its best, and these are not skills that are acquired overnight or indeed by attending an online seminar. The service is sorely in need of midwives with specialist skills.

Despite the impression increasingly given in independent national maternity inquiries and patient surveys, it is unlikely that frontline midwives come to work to ignore women, dismiss their concerns or cause harm to their babies. Of course, there are shameful anecdotes both historical and present day, but most frontline midwives just want to provide the best care they can. Midwifery has always been a great and noble profession, but changes in training and practice have meant that in today's NHS maternity service many midwives feel inadequately trained, increasingly inexperienced (Penna 2024), poorly supported, underconfident, conflicted, out of their depth, professionally vulnerable, mistreated, undervalued or just plain exhausted.

In 2021, the RCM warned of a 'midwifery exodus' following the results of a survey that reported 57 per cent of midwives and midwifery support workers were considering leaving their roles, 84 per cent were concerned about staffing levels, 67 per cent felt the quality of care they deliver is compromised, 54 per cent did not feel valued by their employer and 92 per cent did not feel valued by the government (RCM 2021). And with robust evidence linking poor midwifery staffing levels to increased risk of harmful incidents (Turner et al 2024), it is clear that there is no greater priority than addressing the midwifery staffing crisis.

Frontline obstetrics

Training

The aim of specialist training in obstetrics and gynaecology (O&G) is to create a skilled and competent professional worthy of taking on the responsibility of a woman's reproductive healthcare. Some 30 years ago, postgraduate training was characterised by self-sacrifice, resilience, gruelling timetables and a bizarre degree of reverence towards seniors. The hierarchy was pyramidal; training was a process of elimination. Entry to the bottom rung was marked by introduction to the 'consultant firm'. This was no more than the outgoing senior house officer handing over the pager with a cheery 'there you go'. Clinical guidelines were a pocket-sized *vade mecum* carried around with you in the days of wearing white coats. On-call rotas required 24-hour presence every third or, if you were lucky, every fourth day, with internal cover between juniors for any leave. Shifts lasted up to 72 hours, so there was no prospect of kicking clinical problems into the long grass or adopting the 'wait for the next shift to sort it out' option.

Junior doctors learnt to work efficiently and clear the decks fast. Training posts were appointed for six-month stints and based entirely on references from the consultant. Consultant firms were like a family, a tight-knit group inextricably bound to each other; you liked some members, others not so much. If you got a 'bad' firm, you had to 'suck it up' and hope the next one would be better. On-call rooms were either freezing cold or lacked ventilation. The good ones had torn carpets, a toilet and maybe even a shower. One even had a refrigerator, but it had not worked for years so it was converted into a bookcase. Thankfully, hardly any time was spent in these miserable rooms before the pager erupted again. Busy shifts did not allow for visits to the staff canteen; juniors made do with unused meals from the patient's food trolley. Seriously ill mothers may have secured the attention of the registrar but not usually the senior registrar, who had their own concerns in the pre-consultant years.

Consultants represented the top of the pyramid and were there only in name, a name typically written above the patient's bed on a wipe-clean piece of laminated paper. They appeared on scheduled ward rounds or operating sessions. Prior to the consultant ward round, the registrar would do a frenzied sweep of the patients. Looking foolish might affect progression to the senior registrar grade, which was the biggest career bottleneck at the time. Teaching ward rounds meant bedside presentations and medical students usually took the first blow. Juniors were teased if they hesitated or the registrar had to step in and save them. Senior registrars typically stood around looking smug as juniors dug themselves into a hole. Sometimes the teasing was playful, often not. Some consultants were famous for reducing juniors to tears but mostly juniors were overlooked until they got something wrong. Operating days meant intense and prolonged exposure to the consultant. A standard gynaecology all-day operating list would include a minimum of four major operations, four minor operations and any other acute cases admitted the night before. Operating on 10–12 patients per day was standard practice and the adage 'see one, do one, teach one' reigned supreme. Chatting between cases was initiated by the consultant and usually involved laughing at his (there were very few female consultants) jokes. Much of the work was repetitive and dull – copying out blood results, administering intravenous medication, inserting catheters. The deal was simple; everyone understood the terms of engagement. The weak or half-hearted had to go. I recall one ward round after which the consultant turned to my fellow junior doctor and said, 'Perhaps by Monday you might have thought of an alternate career. I'm sure there is something out there for you, but it isn't O&G.' This was called 'career advice' back then.

Survival meant having each other's backs. Cross-cover for annual leave, study leave, bereavement, getting married, even having a baby was sorted by mutual agreement and kept below the radar of the consultant and ward sister. They were not to be troubled by such 'trivial' matters. Independence and free thinking were encouraged; handholding was for the feeble. Praise was given only for achieving those things not considered part of your job, such as submitting articles for publication or applying for research grants. Such successes resulted in consultant support for undertaking travelling fellowships or exchange visits to other educational establishments. You would jump at the chance, if only to escape the monotony of everyday work and leave the hospital for more than a few hours. RCOG membership exam success earned you a nod from the consultant at the beginning of the next ward round, perhaps even being called by your name. It was worth his while remembering your name now. Exam failure attracted minor sympathy but really it marked you out as a struggler destined for a lesser career. The consultant need not bother learning *your* name: you were not going to make the grade. When you finally became a senior registrar, you were already fully trained to perform clinical duties. This was the easy part done; there were other skills to learn now. Diplomacy, keeping the peace, acting as a bridge between junior colleagues, from whom you were now distancing yourself slowly but surely, and the consultants, whose ranks you hoped to join imminently. The politics of hierarchy could be messy and getting it wrong risked losing support from senior consultants; you were not at the top of the pyramid yet.

There is no doubt that the system was deeply unfair: top jobs in renowned teaching hospitals were given primarily to white Caucasian males, while women got jobs in district general hospitals, despite often being more academically able than their male colleagues. Ethnic minority trainees whose undergraduate training was completed abroad were often appointed to staff grade or associate specialist positions, despite the service being heavily reliant on their clinical experience. Many at the time argued that conditions, working hours and treatment of trainees were inhumane. There were calls for nepotism and favouritism to be abolished in favour of a level playing field. In maternity care, there was a particular backlash against the patriarchy, whose days were clearly numbered. Momentum for change was building, and in 1996 Kenneth Calman, the chief medical officer for England, introduced 'run-through' training, a columnar rather than pyramidal system (HMSO 1993). Finally, an end to the pyramidal process of elimination.

The new training programme brought with it new job titles. Junior and senior house officers were now called foundation year trainees and registrars and senior registrars were renamed specialist registrars, with years of training numbered from 1 to 7. Progression was unrelated to super-curricular achievements, and the absence of bottlenecks meant one could cycle through the system and fall off the end into a consultant post without any experience in allied clinical specialities, research or working abroad. These were considered optional extras. Trainees were to be mentored by named consultants, whose supervisory roles became more formalised. Assessments would be objective, and consultants would have to know their trainees' names if only to log into the correct file on the trainees database. Consultants too got new titles – educational supervisor, training programme director, college tutor. Flow charts with diagrammatic representations of the new system were circulated. Protected study leave was guaranteed so that trainees could prepare for postgraduate exams. In the spirit of fairness, the one-way assessment of trainees by consultants was replaced with 360° assessments in which anyone could grade everyone on everything. Trainees were encouraged to comment anonymously on the quality of their teaching and make suggestions for improvements. Working hours were reduced so that no shift lasted longer than 24 hours and there was a mandatory 12-hour rest period between shifts. At last, a training programme that was more flexible, fair and yes, wait for it... more 'fit for purpose', the purpose presumably still being to create a skilled and competent professional worthy of taking on the responsibility of a woman's reproductive healthcare.

At the time, most, certainly not all, welcomed these reforms, and further changes in postgraduate training became unstoppable. Recent changes mean the word 'trainee' is discouraged in favour of 'lifelong learner' and more and more specialist modules are available, including many non-clinical options. Every time a lifelong learner starts a new rotation, there is a three- to five-day trust induction, during which all routine departmental work is suspended. They are furnished with an inexhaustible supply of online tools and clinical guidelines. Shift lengths have been further reduced to 12 hours, while labour ward shifts are even shorter, with handovers occurring every few hours to pass information from morning to afternoon to evening to overnight shifts. On-call rooms have disappeared because with no shift lasting more than 12 hours doctors can go home to shower and sleep. The emphasis on work–life balance, in combination with the European working time directive first introduced in 2004, dominates NHS workforce strategy today. Attendance on days off or staying behind after a shift to review postoperative patients, or to see interesting cases, is no longer the norm. Juniors, now called 'resident doctors', increasingly 'work to rule' and supervisors are now fearful of negative feedback if they encourage working beyond contracted hours. In addition, as more women have entered the medical profession generally, and O&G in particular, requests for part-time work have increased and for them postgraduate training is taking longer to complete.

In the same way that Project 2000 did not address the problems of midwifery staffing, so run-through training has not addressed the problems of postgraduate training in obstetrics. Chaotic timetables have resulted in infrequent interactions with a range of different consultants, poor exposure to operating theatre sessions and virtually no continuity of care for patients. The impact of run-through training became apparent within only a few years, with surgical trainees reporting less than 50 per cent of operative experience compared to their predecessors (Elbadrawy 2008), a problem replicated in gynaecology (Galvin et al 2023). Junior doctors are no longer apprentices learning from their more experienced seniors, they are shift workers with a different mindset. Clinical problems are allowed to drift from one shift to another and productivity has plummeted. An oft-quoted criticism of the 'old style' training programmes was that it was all about service, with no protected training time, as if it were somehow possible to separate the two, but today's postgraduates have the worst of both worlds – limited exposure to training opportunities and the same, if not worse, pressure to fill service commitments. And although consultants might know the trainees' names, they have no sense of their level of competency because they do not see them regularly. The absence of the consultant firm structure leaves many trainees with no sense of belonging and consultants feeling unmotivated to teach. The consultant reference no longer matters. Instead, postgraduate training is assessed objectively using software packages containing a list of modules with tick-box exercises. Educational supervisors are tasked with signing off on clinical competencies for trainees they may see no

more than a handful of times. Competencies are marked as completed/
not yet completed or on a scale of 1 to 5, in the same way as you might
rate a restaurant or hotel you visited recently.

Both trainers and trainees have expressed reservations about
this style of assessment, but it seems we are stuck with it (rcog.org.
uk/careers-and-training/starting-your-og-career/specialty-training/
assessment-and-progression-through-training). Not only are trainers
unable to provide career advice, they are also disincentivised from
raising serious concerns about a trainee's suitability to progress to the
next level of training, for fear of being accused of being dismissive,
unsupportive or prejudiced. An experienced colleague gave up his
role as an educator due to the frustration of having to allow for
endless second, third even fourth chances because he felt that this
approach would do trainees 'no favours in the end'. Postgraduate
teaching today is formulaic and dull. An in-depth and analytical
approach to clinical practice, based on a solid grounding in anatomy,
physiology and pathology, has been replaced by the rote learning
of the latest nationally agreed guidelines. A wider understanding of
the craftsmanship required to become a mentally agile and dextrous
clinician is no longer required. Ambitious trainees are guilted into
thinking they are selfish, letting down their colleagues or compounding
rota gaps by undertaking supra-curricular activities, and it is made
clear to them that, while personally fulfilling, these ventures will give
them no leverage when applying for consultant positions.

Many postgraduates and younger consultants will no doubt object
to this description. While few could argue that they have comparable
practical experience, most will point to the softer skills they have
that the older generation lacked: good communication, empathy and
inclusiveness. The world is a kinder place, and maternity services
should reflect this. Today, staff are encouraged to be less judgemental,
more accommodating and more accepting of providing care according
to patient wishes and ideals, which makes the ongoing criticisms that
the service fails to listen to its users quite perplexing. Social matters
are given equal priority to medical aspects of care. The younger
generation of frontline workers look dimly upon their seniors who
focused mainly on practical aspects of caregiving and endured abuse
without objection and wonder why they did not call it out. They see

their role as obstetricians as offering information, choice and working in partnership with patients and midwives in that 'everyone matters and is equally important' way much favoured by modern society and commonly referred to as 'flattening the hierarchy'.

All of which is fine until it goes wrong. Then serious questions arise. Where was the chain of command? What should have been done? Who is responsible for the failings? Many obstetricians appear shocked when they realise that comments such as 'But I followed the guidelines' or 'I did the best I could once the midwife called me into the room' or 'I acted in accordance with the mother's wishes' do not constitute a robust defence in the face of a poor outcome. They seem ill prepared to deal with the questions that follow – 'Did you not foresee the problem?' or 'Why did you not offer caesarean delivery sooner?' They take it personally when the mother raises a complaint against them or suggests that they 'failed to inform' her correctly or 'failed to discuss the risks and benefits of all available options'. It is only then that they realise we are most definitely not 'all in it together'. They feel demoralised, deflated, isolated and, yes... guilty. They are less able to deal with the sheer weight of responsibility the job requires. By the time they have learnt the most valuable lesson of all, namely that real 'leadership' (much more about this word later) is all about taking *clinical* responsibility, my observation is that it is often too late. Many will start doubting their clinical acumen and double-checking all their decisions; they feel easily threatened and become increasingly paranoid. Sometimes, this results in defensive practice, distrust of colleagues, lack of participation, deflection of responsibility, avoidance of clinical work, moving to non-patient-facing roles or leaving the service altogether.

Now, I understand why one might think that there was nothing attractive about the training programmes of yesteryear, but many of a certain generation will claim that the means justified the end. If the aim was to become a skilled and competent professional worthy of taking on the responsibility of a woman's reproductive healthcare, then you were part of a system that all but guaranteed it. The hostile elements considered so abhorrent today had a purpose. The practice of medicine is not always straightforward: doctors face intellectual, physical, emotional and ethical challenges daily. They work under constant pressure and are not allowed to have a bad day because there are no second chances. Mistakes cost lives. In obstetrics, the very youngest lives are at stake and the pressure is indescribably immense. When mistakes or complications occur, as they inevitably will from time to time, obstetricians need the resolve to deal with them and continue caring for other patients despite these setbacks. The modern-day obstetrician, through no fault of their own, is less able to deal with these challenges. The current 35-hour working week with only two thirds of the time dedicated to clinical work, while advantageous in other ways, does not allow for similar clinical exposure as the 70+ hour working week of old. And given the five- to seven-year training programme, it would take more than ten years *after* appointment as a consultant to achieve a similar level of clinical experience as the previous generation at the time of their appointment. For routine cases, competence could be achieved sooner, but what of the complex cases?

The job

The aim of postgraduate training is to achieve a consultant post. In the past, neither patients nor juniors expected consultants to provide constant clinical input. They were there to provide clinical leadership, advise on complex cases and further develop the service. Other than a select few equally well-respected senior midwives, no one called them directly without going through the senior registrar first. Senior registrars were expected to have a sixth sense as to the consultant's whereabouts and know the telephone number of his favourite restaurant in the days before mobile phones. At Christmas, consultants invited their firm to their homes for drinks, supper or even a singalong. During summer holidays, there might be a team barbecue. Most consultants were male, so sparring with male juniors by challenging them to a game of golf or tennis was common. Female registrars were invited to join consultants' wives at a book signing or art exhibitions. Today, this would seem pompous posturing, misogynistic or even sexist; back then it was called 'looking after the team'. Consultants were rarely expected to be present out of hours, so they were free to attend their children's concerts or graduation, or pursue hobbies and outside interests. They had paid their dues as trainees, and now it was time to reap the rewards. In retrospect, many considered those days not so miserable after all – the camaraderie was excellent: a best man, godparents to your children or holiday companions were often selected from your training cohort. These strong bonds of friendship were based on trust and mutual respect, admittedly often among like-minded people.

Contrast that with today's consultant – learning on the job, constantly on edge, checking decisions against the latest clinical guidelines, fearful of criticism, poorly supported by peers, little if any control over the working timetable due to staff shortages and often working on split sites with limited opportunities for continuity of care, building teams and establishing supportive relationships. The pressure to provide a consultant-delivered rather than 'just' a consultant-led service is relentless. Junior midwives often bypass the trainees and call consultants directly; mobile phones have made this easy. Postgraduate trainees pass by like ships in the night: there are three, sometimes more, handovers in a 24-hour period. There are steady streams of emails from management containing various directives, increasing numbers of patient complaints and mountains of online paperwork. Clinics often run late, which results in a string of cancelled social engagements. While trainees can work to rule, consultants often feel obliged to stay back and get the work done or 'act down' to cover junior doctors' absences or strikes.

The consultant job many dreamed of has turned out to be a bit of a nightmare, while national inquiry after national inquiry denigrates the service they are nominally in charge of. As consultants today work harder and harder to achieve less and less, so other options begin to look more attractive. For example, the increasingly popular one-way flow towards gynaecology with its reduced out-of-hours commitments has resulted in a two-tier system, in which older, more experienced consultants do mainly daytime gynaecology, leaving younger, less experienced ones to shoulder the unattractive out-of-hours obstetric workload. Older consultants talk openly about 'dumping' obstetric sessions onto newly appointed colleagues, resulting in a lack of available senior clinicians on site during office hours, a notable finding in independent national inquiries. The dominance of females in the speciality makes gender comparisons nowadays virtually obsolete, but sadly the ethnic divisions persist, with non-white colleagues often having less attractive job plans. Controversially, other specialities have engaged physician associates to do the routine work and time will tell if maternity does the same. Yesteryear's inequalities (and make no mistake there were plenty) endure, but the advantages (these were plentiful too) of that bygone era are nowhere to be seen.

The role of a consultant obstetrician in today's NHS maternity service is regarded by many as so unattractive that attrition rates among postgraduate trainees have remained persistently high at around 30 per cent (RCOG 2022), and there is a concerning trend towards early retirement in seniors (RCOG 2020). Interestingly, surveys suggest that the reasons vary with younger doctors leaving due to exhaustion and lack of professional resilience and more senior doctors leaving due to loss of professional identity. Although not as pressing an issue as midwifery staffing, these observations are unsettling.

The overlooked

Inevitably, I have concentrated on midwives and obstetricians but, in my opinion, national inquiries and workforce reports have not placed nearly enough emphasis on other key frontline staff. There are many, but two roles stand out above all because it is impossible to provide a safe maternity service without them.

Anaesthetists

Failure to include this vital speciality in national maternity safety strategies is a grave omission. In the NHS England 'Getting It Right First Time' (GIRFT) report of 2021 on maternity and gynaecology (Richmond & Sherwin 2021), the anaesthetic service is mentioned only twice, almost as an afterthought, although granted it has finally received due recognition in the Maternity Incentive Scheme (2025). There is no such thing as a significant obstetric emergency in which anaesthetic input is not required, so overlooking their contribution is absurd. Those with 'lived experience' of the frontline will know that the second question to ask when you take over a labour ward shift is 'Who is our anaesthetist today?'

Many service users think anaesthetists are there in a supportive role to provide regional analgesia to the 60 per cent or so of women who request this for pain relief in labour. But they are also critical in any operative vaginal delivery (12 per cent), elective caesarean section (18 per cent), emergency caesarean section (21 per cent), obstetric haemorrhage (5 per cent) and severe pre-eclampsia (1–2 per cent – NHS Digital 2023). So, not really a peripheral speciality at all. Without them the obstetrician alone is powerless.

Neonatologists

Neonatology is one of the most expensive services any hospital can provide, so not surprisingly, over the past few decades, there has been a shift towards centralising specialist neonatal care to a handful of units providing care in cases of extreme prematurity, congenital cardiac disease, genetic syndromes, surgical cases and so on. While economically justifiable, this policy has had two problematic consequences. First, it has resulted in many babies being transferred between units either *in utero* (prior to delivery) or *ex utero* in potentially unstable clinical conditions. Second, it has meant that many so-called 'low-risk' units are left with relatively inexperienced neonatal staff, especially out of hours, as more experienced staff are deployed to specialist centres. However, most *unexpected* admissions to special care baby units are term babies who may be very acutely unwell following complicated labours and deliveries. In cases of birth asphyxia and hypoxic ischaemic encephalopathy, which can lead to cerebral palsy, focus is often placed on midwifery and obstetric care, but equally important is the resuscitation and management of the newborn in the first few minutes and hours of life. This is often overlooked or assumed to have been adequate when cases are investigated, and the quality of neonatal care provided at delivery is barely mentioned in most independent national maternity inquiries. Sadly, incident investigations and medicolegal cases have demonstrated that the presence of a competent and experienced neonatologist available exactly when needed, and not a moment later, is crucial. In neonatal resuscitation, every second counts. Attempts at improving maternity care cannot exclude neonatologists from the safety debate, although with limited resources the solutions are unlikely to be easy.

The invisible others

Maternity services cannot run without the help of many other frontline staff, including antenatal screening coordinators responsible for counselling women in relation to a range of investigations, laboratory staff who process test results, sonographers who have the key role in fetal imaging and prenatal diagnoses, ward clerks who coordinate admissions and update patient records, maternity support workers whose input frees up midwives to provide better care, canteen staff who provide refreshments and nutrition to service users, domestic staff who keep the environment clean and safe, and porters who ensure transfers of patients and goods from one area to another. Any service that fails to invest in these individuals and support them in their roles will continue having problematic outcomes.

Conclusion

In the current climate, it is easy for frontline staff working in maternity care to see themselves as downtrodden, devalued lowly shift workers. I would be lying if I said I did not regularly feel this way myself, which often comes as a surprise to trainees who equate seniority with agency. However, we must not despair as there is much that could be improved if the following issues are addressed:

+ Admit that accelerated training programmes based on 'tick-box' exercises are not a substitute for clinical exposure.
+ Opportunities and support for frontline staff to further their careers in the *clinical* arena are vital at both a personal and a service level. Failure to do so means frontline staff will continue to look elsewhere to achieve this.
+ Safe practice means working within strong, stable teams and such teams are not built overnight. Mentorship is crucial and requires the physical presence of senior midwives and obstetricians.
+ The priorities of frontline workers should always be clinical. That is not to say that patients' social and psychological wellbeing is unimportant, but when judgements come, which they will, it is clinical performance that matters most.
+ Frontline staff should be transparent about what proportion of

their work is clinical versus non-clinical, and the value of any activity undertaken that does not directly help them look after patients should be scrutinised.

✦ Most shifts are completed without adverse events because frontline staff manage to spread themselves so thin that they cover all the work, often at considerable personal cost. If we want long-term, workable solutions, frontline workers need to keep raising staffing concerns, even in the absence of poor outcomes.

✦ Frontline staff must recognise that although their work can be frustrating, off-the-cuff comments or certain behaviours can come across as dismissive and cause reputational damage to individuals and organisations. Although interpretation varies greatly, words have lasting impact.

✦ The public must be made aware that strike action is not simply about remuneration; it reflects the much deeper concerns of frontline staff about the value placed upon them as manifested through the working environment, availability of equipment and their treatment by others, and is an expression of genuine worry for the future of their profession.

✦ While independent national inquiries focus on training and healthcare processes, and more recently place the service users interests front and centre of the reports, the opinions and challenges faced by frontline staff are largely overlooked. Their stories must be told because they are in a much more powerful position than they might think, for two reasons. First, they are ideally placed to identify both the enablers of and the obstacles to good care and, second, they are 'the doers'. Without them there simply *is no Service*.

But it is impossible to look at frontline staff in isolation. In the next chapter, I will turn my attention to the second of the three main stakeholders in NHS maternity care – managers, who are the service organisers.

4 Service organisers – management in maternity care

Introduction

The NHS is often framed as a service in which nurses and doctors are responsible for providing care, assisted by managers working in the background to organise the service according to changes in demand. In this chapter, I describe how management in maternity care has changed over the past 30 years and what drivers have shaped the service we have today.

The maternity management of old

As I outlined in Chapter 2, before the establishment of the NHS in 1948, maternity care was primarily a community-based, midwifery-led service supported by general practitioners. Unwell mothers were admitted to lying-in hospitals founded and funded by the middle and upper classes (Cody 2004). Many of these buildings still survive today and their facades often tell the stories of their past. These institutions appointed an almoner, typically a middle-class woman whose job was to assess each patient's social standing, family circumstances and ability to pay, and fees were levied accordingly. A visiting physician or surgeon or surgeon accoucheur would work with a senior nurse or midwife to oversee the general running of the unit. The management team was comprised of this small group of experienced clinicians in charge of a larger team of nurses, midwives and orderlies who provided minute-to-minute care, and each unit functioned autonomously.

In 1948, things were about to change. The government commissioned a review of maternity services culminating in the Cranbrook report in 1959, which recommended that 70 per cent of births should take place in hospital, with 30 per cent at home only if approved by an obstetrician. In 1970, the Peel Report took it one step further and recommended that all women deliver in hospital because this was safer and, despite some opposition, this was an easy win because by that time less than 5 per cent of women were delivering at home. Thus, within 25 years of the foundation of the NHS, maternity had switched from being a community-based midwifery-led service to a hospital-based one.

Accommodating births in hospital settings alongside general expansion of other NHS services necessitated ongoing reform and adaptation to the previous rudimentary management structure, and inevitably administrative processes became more complex (The King's Fund 2010). Local community appointed almoners were replaced by NHS managers who were expected to keep abreast of matters related to finances, schedule clinical events, procure consumables and ensure maintenance of equipment and estates. These managers were not clinicians, so they relied upon input from the same small group of nurses, midwives and doctors, typically senior staff who undertook these advisory roles as a goodwill gesture towards a department they had worked in for many years. They would attend management meetings from time to time, outline the needs of their department and, following discussion with their frontline colleagues, proffer opinions as to how best to address them. It was the job of the managers to listen, understand the issues and action the necessary changes. This system worked because the requirements of service users were identified by frontline staff and a clinical representative acted as a messenger to convey this information to managers who allocated resources accordingly.

Inevitably, there were minor tweaks to this arrangement as time went on, but the 1980s saw a seismic step change in management style within the NHS. At that time, management strategies were evolving rapidly in the business sector and attempts to mirror this in healthcare were considered visionary (Griffiths Report 1983). Over the next decade, two new revolutionary concepts were introduced and notwithstanding several name changes and reincarnations, a recurrent theme in NHS management, they still dominate all aspects of the NHS today – 'healthcare commissioning' and 'healthcare regulation'. I will explain these two guiding principles in some detail because they are key to how the NHS functions (or malfunctions) today, and without an understanding of them the rest of this book will not make sense.

Establishing the new order
Healthcare commissioning

In January 1989, the White Paper, 'Working for patients (NHS reforms)', proposed a clear division between purchasers and providers of healthcare, with GP fundholders acting as purchasers of the state-funded health services provided in secondary and tertiary care settings, ie specialist clinics and hospitals. This required new contracts to be drawn up for GPs and hospital doctors, which was done in April 1990. Two months later, the National Health Service and Community Care Act 1990 was passed and the new internal market became a reality. It was hoped that these changes would give GPs purchasing power and the opportunity to offer their patients choice and improved efficiency. Providers were tasked with creating responsive and competitive hospital-based services using budgets devolved to NHS trusts and individual directorates within them.

In this brave new world of healthcare commissioning, it soon became clear that continued provision of clinical services was dependent upon careful control of the allocated budget. Much time, effort and expense was spent on setting tariffs such that, even though the public was not expected to pay for care directly out of their pockets, the financial value of every patient encounter, investigation, procedure or prescription had to be quantified. Over the decades 'purchasers' have been called GP fundholders, primary care trusts, clinical commissioning groups (CCGs) and, following the publication of the Health and Social Care Act 2022, which aimed to pull away from this transactional model of healthcare towards a collaborative multi-service partnership model, renamed integrated care groups (ICGs) or integrated care boards (ICBs). Despite ever softer nomenclature, the central role of commissioners remains to ensure providers price their service competitively and demonstrate value for money (Wenzel et al 2023). Trusts are now run like businesses, employing branding experts and adopting straplines and mission statements. Letterheads and email sign-offs are tagged with logos and motivational messages, each trust claiming to be more kind, welcoming, caring, visionary, specialised, innovative, friendly, inclusive, diverse, expert and understanding than the other. Frontline staff are expected to act in accordance with trust values and managers to provide proof of this.

I recall my first encounter with the new style of tariff-obsessed manager. It was 1994 and she was a nurse by training, in her late forties and holding a clipboard. I recall feeling uncomfortable as she invited herself onto the ward round, and even more alarmed when she stood far too close to the cubicle curtains as I went to examine a woman undergoing induction of labour for pre-eclampsia. As I emerged, she asked what I had done – was it just an abdominal examination or a vaginal examination too? Did I request fetal monitoring? Or change the mother's antihypertensive medication? How long was she likely to be in hospital? Every action was noted down on her clipboard. To me, the patient was a woman having a baby, with both needing close monitoring as this was a high-risk case. To her, the patient was Bed 12, followed by a series of coded numbers. This basic pen and paper coding system was to evolve into a series of ever more complex electronic systems. The NHS now employs thousands of coders who sit in back offices trawling through patient records assigning codes to various aspects of care. In theory, these coding systems provide data upon which future service provision can be planned but their main purpose is reimbursement, even though it is widely acknowledged that they are deeply flawed and much of the data collected is meaningless (O'Dowd 2010; CHKS 2014).

Healthcare regulation

Even from the outset, it was recognised that the public would not accept services being commissioned on their behalf based on competitive pricing and punchy straplines alone, so the extra dimension of 'clinical safety' had to be included. This was formalised by way of the Citizen's

Charter in 1991, which stressed the role of the patients as 'customers' who had the right to expect and receive not only competitively priced care but care that was of the highest 'quality' delivered 'efficiently'. But what did these vague terms mean? The pressure was on to find ways of measuring 'quality' and 'efficiency', and this resulted in the introduction of vast swathes of clinical 'targets'. In 1994, provider performance tables were published for the first time, and this allowed 'purchasers' and 'customers' to compare units. This revealed significant disparities in the quality of clinical services, and in 1997 the White Paper – 'The new NHS: modern, dependable' – acknowledged that the standard of care in the NHS was variable and the service was slow to respond to lapses in quality. It was widely agreed that decisions regarding ongoing provision of clinical services should not be left to commissioners, who had their eyes primarily on the money, but instead more overarching quality control systems were needed to standardise care nationally (Walshe, 2002; Lewis, 2006).

In 1999, the Commission for Healthcare Improvement (CHI) was established with the purpose of assisting NHS hospitals in implementing standardised and safe care. Hospitals and residential and domiciliary care settings would in turn submit themselves to regular inspections by the newly established National Standards Commission (NSC), responsible for assessing whether organisations adhered to safety standards and had relevant staff training in place. The CHI and NSC merged in 2003 to form the Healthcare Commission (HCC), which became the Care Quality Commission (CQC) in 2009. From 2010, all facilities providing healthcare in England were legally obliged to register with the CQC and agree to regular inspections. As with its predecessors, the aim of the CQC was, in theory, to provide guidance on how to meet standards of safety and protect the public from harm associated with substandard care. With time, commissioning groups, sensitive to the criticism that they were only willing to support 'cheap' services, got in on the act and they too started demanding safety and efficiency data from providers, so trust management teams were put under the spotlight by both healthcare commissioners and healthcare regulators. In practice, healthcare regulation was achieved by appointing a mobile army of auditors who scored completed tasks in a binary fashion, the endpoint being a mechanically generated overall verdict.

Although there were league tables and comparative performance guides in operation previously, notably for acute care and ambulance services, it was in 2001 that the NHS introduced the formal 'star rating' system. Ratings were awarded following inspections, and scoring well required providers to demonstrate compliance with key targets related to cleanliness, waiting times, a range of clinical and non-clinical services and patient feedback. The star rating system was later replaced with a four-point scale – outstanding, good, requires improvement and inadequate. League tables and ratings have never been popular with frontline staff because many feel they are awarded based on targets which correlate poorly with clinical outcomes. Nevertheless, with these metrics now in place, NHS management teams were incentivised to ensure their units performed well, and it soon became clear that the culture of target-driven care was here to stay. Many targets were set locally, others regionally and the most important targets, such as A&E waiting times or cancer referral pathways, were set nationally. Breaching targets was, and still is, penalised by poor trust ratings, adverse media coverage, cessation of funding, withdrawal of the service or unit closure.

Healthcare commissioning and healthcare regulation in practice

Over the past three decades, the pressure placed on service organisers to action financially driven ways of working and meet nationally agreed compliance targets in relation to service safety and efficiency has resulted in three phenomena:

1) Expansion of NHS management

Adhering to the increasing demands set out by commissioners and regulators has required uncompromising and relentless expansion of management teams but, curiously, it is surprisingly difficult to determine just how much taxpayers' money is spent on this. Official NHS workforce data is confusing but suggests that somewhere between 2 and 4 per cent of all NHS staff are employed in a management role. In fact, this figure most likely represents the 'real' managers who are not clinicians by training. The NHS cannot afford the salaries the very best managers can attract in the corporate sector, so these managers need assistance from people with clinical backgrounds. This trend of encouraging clinical staff to take on managerial roles started in the early 1990s and has snowballed since. Now here is the trick. These individuals remain on clinical contracts and clinical pay scales, so as far as NHS human resources databases are concerned, they do not factor into the 2–4 per cent headcount; instead they continue to be regarded as 'clinicians'. In other hybrid roles within healthcare, there are systems for pro rata payment. For example, clinical academics who hold honorary clinical contracts might have 50 per cent of their salary paid by an NHS trust (patient-facing work) and the other 50 per cent from the medical school, charitable foundation or research grant awarding body (academic work). This makes it easy to determine what proportion of time such an individual spends attending to patients' healthcare needs and what proportion is spent ensconced in a laboratory or lecture theatre. But the salaries of so-called 'clinical managers' are unformulated and, given the pressures to comply with an ever-expanding list of management directives, it is easy to see how clinical commitments are squeezed out of their timetables. In my experience, these changes often creep up on them insidiously with many not recognising the metamorphosis that has occurred, leaving many still fervently believing their primary role is clinical.

Those outside the health profession might wonder why individuals who have worked hard to acquire degrees in nursing or medicine might choose to do management jobs. Well, there are three reasons for this. First, a sad indictment of the modern NHS is that the only way to advance your career is to take on such roles. In nursing and midwifery, it is impossible to progress to a higher pay scale without taking on management responsibilities and placement on the highest bands often means 'pure' management. This is also increasingly true for doctors. For example, clinical excellence awards, historically the domain of medical academics, are now mainly given to individuals involved in management, although their efforts are often packaged as quality improvement or innovation activities to give them a veneer of clinical credibility. Second, given how stressful and thankless frontline work in maternity care is, managerial roles offer an altogether better quality of life and the opportunity of working within a large and well-supported team. Despite notional out-of-hours commitments written into some maternity manager roles, most are essentially 9–5 jobs and, in the post-Covid era, largely involve working from home. Third, the limited resources available to appoint more frontline staff do not apply to positions in management. A new management role can be suggested, approved, job planned, advertised and appointed within a matter of weeks, whereas for frontline staff, especially senior doctors, it can take several months or even years.

I believe this drifting of clinically trained frontline maternity staff into management roles explains, at least in part, why service users do not feel that the increases in numbers of midwives and doctors often reported in the media or boasted of by politicians are real. These people exist; they are just not working on the frontline, so they are never 'seen'. The taxpayer does pay for them, but exactly how much remains unknown.

We know that about 45 per cent of the total NHS budget of around £200 billion per annum is spent on 'staff' salaries. According to The King's Fund, in February 2024 there were 140,700 doctors, 377,600 nursing staff and 39,800 managers out of a total workforce of 1.34 million, making the number of managers 2.9 per cent of the total. Between 2011 and 2024, the number of doctors increased by 45 per cent, nurses by 26 per cent and managers by 18 per cent (The King's Fund 2024). This apparently modest number of managers has led some analysts to argue that the NHS is undermanaged rather than overmanaged (Kirkpatrick & Malby 2022). But there is no data to reveal the proportion of clinicians' time spent bolstering the activity of the 'real' managers.

2) The obsession with data

Continued funding of a service is contingent upon favourable data relating to expenditure, productivity and compliance. Collecting, inputting, processing, analysing and presenting data is labour intensive, so management teams today have come to resemble the clinical firms of the past with a pyramidal hierarchy: administrators at the bottom, junior managers in the middle and senior managers at the top. Senior managers hold the key to deciding which services are provided, where, when and by whom. Gone are the days of frontline clinician autonomy and ad hoc advice given to a small management team by clinical representatives acting as patient advocates. Such ideals are considered old fashioned and ill suited to the modern-day NHS. Today, clinical services are only provided if supported by a mass of complex, intertwined, often duplicated processes negotiated by managers with managers. Services can be withdrawn with little debate, consideration, time for reflection or recourse to appeal simply because data suggests the service is no longer cost effective or targets have not been met. The bureaucracy is breathtaking and, because resources are limited, the success of one unit is intrinsically linked to failure of another in what has become a bizarre 'winner takes all' war of attrition between providers. The 'competition' so eagerly hailed in the 1990s has not improved care for patients but has rather resulted in a race to the bottom as managers go to battle armed with data to prove their service is more cost effective, less wasteful and more compliant than their rivals'.

3) Mergers and closures

Management teams are obliged to take decisive action when data suggests a unit is 'underperforming'. As a result, mergers and closures have become a fact of everyday life and, while demonstrations and the signing of petitions aimed at keeping various healthcare establishments open have become commonplace, the general public is rarely aware of why some units become earmarked for closure in the first place.

Independent national inquiries into maternity care often highlight growing dissatisfaction and poor morale among frontline staff working in units threatened by mergers or closure. This may seem odd to outsiders, given that NHS staff rarely lose their jobs or suffer pay cuts as a result and, apart from the slight hassle associated with commuting to another (usually nearby) maternity unit, they suffer no tangible consequences. Surely everyone should subscribe to a more efficient, streamlined, less wasteful way of working with pooled resources and an amalgamation of talent? Well, the truth is that frontline staff rarely object to mergers and closures per se; what they object to is how they are enacted in practice and the consequences for patient care.

Typically, the less favoured unit is denuded of resources thus ensuring it falls short on targets, making the victorious unit appear 'better', although in all probability, the favoured unit also has significant problems with staff shortages, inadequate skill mix, rota gaps, insufficient equipment, poor workflows and failing infrastructure, not to mention adverse patient outcomes. Thus, the merger/closure does *not* result in an improved service. In the corporate sector, mergers and closures do not just result in relocation of staff but also a better resourced working environment, enhanced efficiency and productivity, increased revenue, redundancy pay for employees whose skills are no longer needed or those unable or unwilling to transfer, and potentially improved career progression for staff who remain. None of this happens in the NHS, prompting many frontline staff to remark 'same misery, different address'. More importantly, mergers and closures can be dangerous because they force frontline staff to work within unfamiliar teams in unfamiliar settings, changes they know risk tipping the service beyond a critical mass of workload which is challenging but manageable to being overwhelming and thus unsafe.

Small, familiar and stable teams are safe teams. Big, in NHS terms, is definitely not better because economies of scale do not work well in healthcare. Failure to provide continuity of care in maternity has been identified as a key contributor to poor perinatal outcomes, and the need to address this has featured *ad nauseam* in the recommendations of all independent national maternity inquiries for several decades. Yet, during that same time period, the number of maternity units facing mergers and closures has increased with many pregnant women having care split over several sites. Mothers are often sent for delivery to one unit having had all their antenatal care in another. I have even reviewed cases in which mothers were transferred between units in the middle of induction of labour. Reduced capacity means that it is now 'normal' practice to divert women in labour to neighbouring units (Townsend 2024). Frontline staff who raise objections to these practices are often vilified. In one meeting, the head of midwifery explained how 'the younger midwives were coping better' with the recent merger and it was 'just a case of waiting for the older ones to be flushed out of the system' as if these senior staff were excrement. When challenged by a senior ward sister whether this approach might risk loss of experienced midwives, the retort was, 'Midwives are not there to do as they please, they are there to do as they are told.'

Maternity managers – what, who and how?

Now that I have explained the two guiding principles that dictate all aspects of service organisation, I will turn my attention to the individuals who pull at the levers of power.

What do maternity service managers do... in theory?

Organising 'the Service' means addressing each of its three components: people, tools and spaces.

The people part is the most complex. Having identified patients' needs, maternity managers are supposed to recruit staff with the correct skills, promote training and teaching, formulate meaningful job plans, ensure productivity and high standards of work, engender a good work ethic, encourage career development, help staff who experience difficulties, assist in staff appraisal, facilitate transparency and good communication, ensure that disciplinary measures are reasonable and proportionate, assist in the retention of skilled workers, support academic research and innovation, and safeguard against prejudicial treatment.

Other managers oversee the purchasing, upgrading and maintenance of equipment. This involves negotiating with suppliers, keeping a keen eye on stock, understanding changing trends in patient care and being able to map out future demands.

As far as spaces are concerned, the NHS manager's role here is inevitably limited because NHS estates are often under the control of local authorities so changes are often dependent on town planning procedures and central government funding.

Who are the maternity managers?

Broadly speaking, managers fall into two groups. The first and larger group are midwives in the later stages of their career, too young to retire but unkeen to keep working on the frontline due to exhaustion and burnout. They are often biding their time until retirement. Their roles are predominantly administrative and focus on data collection and following administrative processes. Typically, their career goals are limited, they stay working within a given trust, they are dutiful and take instruction well from their 'seniors'. This second group is smaller and senior only in name as they are typically much younger and much more ambitious. A lifetime of being overworked, undermined, disempowered and underpaid was not for them, so they entered management roles early in their careers with meagre clinical experience – although to read their CVs you might not know this. They are not interested in quiet back-office roles because they are not 'just' managers: they consider themselves to be 'leaders' and move comfortably between trusts and other NHS organisations with remarkable regularity.

Obstetricians have joined the managerial ranks in increasing numbers in the past 20 years. A potent catalyst for this migration away from clinical work was the rolling-out of formalised job planning in 2005. This was arguably the nail in the coffin for the medical profession more generally and, among a litany of disastrous unintended consequences, this process gave equal weighting in financial terms to programmed activities whether they were clinical or non-clinical in nature. This meant that managerial duties were no longer undertaken for altruistic reasons but now needed to be taken seriously to justify the remuneration attached to them. Formal job descriptions were drawn up and interviews held to ensure only the committed were appointed.

Not surprisingly, these roles were considered too restrictive to senior consultants who had previously occupied them on a voluntary basis, so many bowed out, opening opportunities for more junior colleagues to get involved. The fact that significant remuneration and a whole lot more kudos could be achieved relatively easily was undoubtedly attractive to this group who, for the reasons I have outlined in Chapter 3, were coping less well with the relentless commitments of clinical work. Operational naivety meant they were more emollient and pliable, so they could be more easily persuaded into pursuing agendas dictated by healthcare commissioners and healthcare regulators without challenging their purposes or anticipating their likely consequences.

Most consultant obstetricians today cannot remember a time before healthcare commissioning and healthcare regulation came to dominate all aspects of service provision, which has resulted in submissive acceptance of any demands placed upon the service by them. Appointment to a consultant job today is conditional upon the applicant being able to demonstrate 'management experience', which might seem a warped priority at a time when the frontline is so depleted. As one insightful postgraduate trainee said to me during an educational supervision meeting, 'We all know you are better off doing a silly little quality improvement project that might save the NHS a few pennies rather than undertaking a secondment to a visionary research unit implementing robotic gynaecological surgery or new ways of fetal imaging.' Sadly, in the modern-day maternity service, honing clinical skills is considered a waste of time, and staff are encouraged to believe that career progression can only be achieved through management.

In keeping with the National Leadership Council's vision of 'world-class leadership talent and leadership development at every level in the NHS' (NHS Institute for Innovation and Improvement 2005), there are no shortages in career development opportunities in NHS management. Although they vary between maternity units, the array of management roles available to aspirational midwives and obstetricians is mind-boggling: supervisor of midwives, practice development midwife, lead for antenatal services, head of community services, head of caseload midwifery, lead for home births, associate head of midwifery, head of midwifery, freedom to speak up champion, senior maternity safety officer, risk management lead, champion for equality and diversity, lead for maternity quality assurance, maternity CQC lead, head of maternity governance and compliance, general manager for women's health, trust divisional director of nursing and midwifery, clinical lead for audit, head of clinical risk management, postgraduate education lead, digital communications lead, data quality lead, obstetric drills training champion, head of speciality, clinical director, deputy clinical director, head of maternity safety strategy, divisional director for maternity, regional lead for maternity.

In many trusts, combined posts in maternity and paediatrics are common, such as lead for women's and children's services. At the highest levels of trust management, associate medical directors, medical directors or even chief executives can be drawn from any medical speciality. It would be natural to assume that many of these jobs involve direct patient care because the titles sound clinical, but that would be a mistake. Anyone who is serious about climbing the NHS management career pathway is required to attend regular training sessions and endless numbers of meetings, and accrue a multitude of management certificates, diplomas or even degrees. Networking is also crucial, so the absence of clinical commitments is a prerequisite to achieving a position in senior management. The requirement for clinically trained staff to do a minimum number of hours of clinical work to maintain professional registration becomes just a formality, an easy sign-off by a fellow manager. In my view, such paltry exposure to patient care is driven by guilt rather than a sense of duty, making some attendances in clinical areas more of a liability than an asset: they are brief, with a back-up 'proper' frontline midwife or obstetrician in place to allow for a quick getaway.

But these appearances are enough to pull the wool over the eyes of everyone at the top of the organisation, such as executive and non-executive directors or even the chair of the trust. These individuals, whose role does not extend to regular visits to the clinical frontline to fact-check, frequently praise senior clinical managers for the great clinical work they continue to do despite their managerial commitments. However, a truly stellar career in NHS management cannot be achieved without regular moves between trusts, resulting in the phenomenon frontline workers are all too familiar with, namely someone from outside who has never worked in the unit suddenly appearing and telling them how to run the show then disappearing a few months later. Better still is moving on to any number of 'external' or 'arm's length' organisations because this takes away the pressures associated with representing or bidding on behalf of a solitary provider. For many decades, these organisations have been created, merged, separated, abolished, revamped, rebranded and renamed by successive governments under the umbrella term of 'NHS management restructuring'.

In practice, this national addiction is simply a teasingly obscure game of deception and confusion that makes it almost impossible to assess the value of any of these organisations or hold their staff to account. At the time of writing, options for maternity managers wishing to immerse themselves in roles within local healthcare commissioning groups involve liaising with CCGs/ICGs/ICBs, although studies have shown that 75 per cent of these groups are failing specifically on maternity care (Gammie 2016). Some become involved in health and wellbeing Boards (HWBs – see local.gov.uk/our-support/partners-care-and-health/care-and-health-improvement/health-and-wellbeing-systems) or other community-based organisations that advise commissioning groups, roles that are often stepping stones to larger national organisations such as the NHS Business Services Authority (nhsbsa.nhs.uk), the organisation responsible for issuing maternity exemption certificates which allow women to obtain free prescriptions and dental care during and for 12 months after pregnancy. Other options include NHS Resolution (NHSR, resolution.nhs.uk), previously called the NHS Litigation Authority (NHSLA), an organisation that investigates claims and purports to play a role in improving care based on lessons learnt. Then there is NHS Blood and Transplant (nhsbt.nhs.uk), which manages blood and organ donation throughout the UK and with national obstetric haemorrhage rates rising (Ahmadzia 2020), maternity representation is welcome.

For those with experience in data collection, a role within NHS Digital (digital.nhs.uk) or its subgroups beckons. These include the Health and Social Care Information Centre or the Maternity Services Data Set, which captures what is referred to as 'patient-level data' extracted from antenatal booking appointments with the aim of reporting, commissioning and monitoring of outcomes and inequalities. For those interested in research, the National Institute for Health Research (nihr.ac.uk) supports a network of investigators by funding projects on hypertensive disorders and prematurity, which, although important, are not necessarily where the worst clinical outcomes occur. Careers in teaching or continuing professional development with organisations such as Health Education England (hee.nhs.uk) or local education and training boards are always popular, although many frontline staff question how it is possible to teach and assess others when not actively involved in clinical practice. Nevertheless, these include the Maternity Safety Training Fund, maternity e-learning, continuity of carer training, expansion of the midwifery training role, and implementation of the Maternity Support Worker Framework, among others.

Some managers will take up advisory roles with the National

Institute for Health and Care Excellence (NICE – nice.org.uk), which provides guidance based on the best available clinical evidence, while others opt for roles in public information and work with Public Health England, established in 2013, but since replaced by the National Institute for Health Protection, the UK Health Security Agency and the Office for Health Promotion. In maternity, the focus is on antenatal screening and promoting advice regarding smoking, alcohol, drugs and vaccines (UK Health Security Agency 2022). Until the announcement of its abolition in March 2025, the most aspirational managers aimed for roles within NHS England (NHSE) (england.nhs.uk/maternity). This organisation (previously known as the NHS Commissioning Board) was established in 2013 after the Health and Social Care Act 2012 recommended the NHS should have operational independence from the government. For many years, NHSE was considered the most influential of all arm's-length bodies because of its role in overseeing many of the previously mentioned organisations and upholding the values and commitments outlined by the NHS constitution in England. Scotland, Wales and Northern Ireland have had equivalent organisations with similar remits. Its abolition will apparently result in a 50 per cent reduction in headcount across NHSE and DHSC which currently employs 18,000, many from 'clinical' backgrounds, albeit not clinically active in practice so the 'job losses for nurses and doctors' that the media have reported is unlikely to be something patients notice. According to the prime minister, Kier Starmer, these changes will bring the NHS more directly under government control, release £500 million for frontline care, prevent NHS frontline staff from 'drowning in micromanagement' and establish a healthcare service with 'fewer checkers and more doers' even if this means taking on 'vested interests' and those who do not want to change the status quo (NHS Confederation 2025).

In practice this is likely to take at least two years, require parliamentary approval and involve a large number of objectors being placated with generous golden handshakes. And in any event, the propensity for these organisations to return under a different but equally wasteful guise should not be underestimated. For example, in 2018, NHSE itself was merged with NHS Improvement, a body responsible for overseeing NHS foundation trusts. NHS Improvement was in turn made up of several smaller organisations such as Monitor and the NHS Trust Development Authority, so these too were abolished upon completion of the merger in 2022, but much of the workforce was absorbed by the new organisation. Also, the 'direct government control' element must be questioned because other organisations such as NHS Providers (nhsproviders.org), a spin-off from NHS Confederation, employ staff who are instrumental in negotiating healthcare provision by trusts with the DHSC. In maternity, at the time of writing there is nothing to suggest that the large number of programmes run by well-staffed subcommittees that NHSE has supported over the years, which aim to promote 'choice and personalised care in maternity services', will be affected. These include the Maternity Transformation Programme; Choice and Personalised Care in Maternity Services; the Maternity Safety Support Programme; the Maternity and Neonatal Safety Improvement Programme (MNSI), previously called Healthcare Safety Investigation Branch (HSIB); National Maternity Data Viewer; Better Births and its related programmes; Improving Equity and Equality in Maternity and Neonatal Care; Maternity Safety Champions; Preventing Avoidable Admission of Term Babies to Special Care; Maternity – Talking Heads; Saving Babies' Lives Care Bundles; and Maternity and Neonatal Voices Partnerships.

Organisations with a particular focus on healthcare regulation are especially keen to see themselves as 'independent', although they all fall under the DHSC umbrella and are taxpayer funded so this seems inexplicable to many. Most healthcare inspectors are ex-NHS managers who, having been at the receiving end of the checklist, are all too familiar with the marking scheme. Thus, the regulatory process, which is supposed to protect patients from harm, has been reduced to a checklist of completed actions in which both the assessor and the assessed know what to do and say in order to pass with flying colours. The Care Quality Commission is the most notable healthcare regulator at the time of writing, and despite ongoing concerns and recent inquiries that have suggested the CQC is not fit for purpose (Darzi 2024), this organisation continues to have considerable reach.

Other regulatory bodies include the Medicines and Healthcare Products Regulatory Agency (gov.uk/government/organisations/medicines-and-healthcare-products-regulatory-agency), which makes sure that medicines and medical devices are safe to use; the Human Tissue Authority (hta.gov.uk), which regulates use of human tissue such as donated organs; and more relevant to our speciality, the Human Fertilisation and Embryology Authority (hfea.gov.uk), which regulates fertility treatments and the use of embryos in research.

Despite being in active clinical practice long before most of these organisations were created, I still have no real sense of why so many are needed and what they have achieved other than serving the career development needs of ambitious managers. Undoubtedly, some of the work managers do both within trusts and the wider external bodies discussed above is needed, but the amount of taxpayers' money involved in funding these roles remains unknown. This should leave many feeling at the very least curious and uncomfortable because every penny spent on service organisation is one less penny spent on service provision.

What do maternity service managers do… in practice?

In the NHS, the success of management teams is predicated upon the fervent belief that implementation of processes dictated by commissioners and regulators will translate into better clinical outcomes despite evidence that these processes are costly without any measurable benefit to patients (Oikonomou et al 2019). Nevertheless, completing tasks requires steely determination and a preoccupation with box ticking that should not be underestimated. It is my observation that many clinical staff who dip their toe into managerial waters do so with honourable intentions but soon falter or find themselves wrestling with their conscience when they realise the stark incompatibility in mindset required to be an effective caregiver versus an effective manager, roles that do not make for comfortable bedfellows. Anyone hoping for an accomplished career in management learns to adapt quickly and revise their priorities or get out.

Adapting quickly means understanding that implementing and measuring processes becomes the main aim; clinical outcomes are incidental byproducts. Data exists as 'proof' that budget boundaries are respected and safety standards met. Extra brownie points and a more accelerated career path await those who can demonstrate cost savings under the various 'cost improvement schemes' or 'transformational change schemes', although official pitches carefully concentrate on issues of maternal choice and clinical safety rather than penny pinching (NHS England 2016; NHSR 2025). The ultimate goal is maintaining, ideally improving, service ratings, a springboard that launches a manager up the career ladder.

The sympathetic view of maternity service organisers is that their roles are thankless, and that the pressures and demands placed upon them are unreasonable and impossible to meet without being unpopular with both frontline workers and service users. The less sympathetic view is that their ascendency to power has in many cases proved to be an insidious and malevolent influence which has led to 'poor unit culture', a phrase that appears recurrently in independent national inquiries. 'Unit culture' is a term used to describe acceptable norms, the unwritten rules as it were, that operate within a workplace, and it encompasses notions of values, ideas, customs, beliefs, dress code, behaviours, rituals, styles of communication and so on. The association between 'poor unit culture' and healthcare failings has long been recognised (Mannion & Davies 2018). Those with the highest profiles within any organisation set the standards. Undoubtedly there are positive examples, but the *modus operandi* of management teams working in maternity units with the most extreme examples of 'poor unit culture' commonly include the following shortcomings:

1. Poor or deceptive communication

Management directives almost always require frontline staff to do something differently or on top of what they are already doing. Foisting even more work upon hard-pressed frontline staff can prove tricky, so communications are brief, usually by email, and often written in the third person: 'It has been decided that…'. Individuals likely to raise eyebrows are often excluded from communications; those less likely or able to object are included under the false pretence of 'canvassing opinion'. Deputies are often sent to meetings where objectors are likely to be present leaving these minions to shield their seniors from awkward and uncomfortable questions. Holidays are often scheduled for the day after a bomb has been dropped thus ensuring uncontactability in the aftermath of an explosion. For the least palatable messages, a favourite tactic is what behavioural psychologists call 'triangulation', in which one thing is said to one group of staff but presented differently to another. This is designed to cause doubt and discomfort and foster fear and tribalism.

Communications are often manipulated to allow for broad inter-pretation of events. For example, 'differences of opinion' means completely opposing priorities and perspectives, 'integrating' or 'redirecting' the service means mergers and closures, 'reallocating resources' means withdrawing funding, 'offering support in a new role' means presenting frontline staff with changes in their job plans that are a *fait accompli*. Failures are often transmuted or rebranded as successes or turned into 'learning points'. For example, being referred for mediation is 'an opportunity to get to know the team better', being subject to a disciplinary is 'taking time to reflect on one's career', or being suspended is 'leaving to focus on the next phase of one's life'. Much to the bewilderment of frontline staff, this sort of language is used effortlessly in progress reports, so it is little wonder that healthcare commissioners and healthcare inspectors often get an unjustifiably rosy impression of units in which there are serious problems. In retrospect, the awarding of favourable ratings and thus ongoing funding makes the assessors feel duped or look foolish when the truth is unearthed, as happened with the investigation into maternity services at Shrewsbury and Telford Hospital NHS Trust.

2. The ability to dissociate power and accountability

If targets are achieved, cost savings made or favourable ratings awarded, managers even peripherally involved in the project will take full credit, acting swiftly to raise their profile within the organisation. Actions include a valedictory lap around the department bearing the CQC's 'outstanding' banner or photo opportunities issuing 'worker of the week' certificates. Pictures in trust newsletters of managers looking relaxed while doing walkabouts on wards provide evidence of 'mentorship', 'leadership' and 'visibility', words that appear on healthcare inspectors' checklists.

In contrast, criticism is to be sidestepped and failures need to be hidden or deflected. Big teams make this easier because individual managers can claim that they 'knew nothing', their 'hands were tied' or the problem was 'outside [their] remit'. Most problems can be buried under the mountain of dirt called 'under investigation'. Internal investigations are time consuming and can be further delayed by deliberate obfuscation so that by the time recommendations are finally made the management team has been 'restructured', senior individuals within it have moved on, and everyone else has forgotten the issues raised in the first place. Sometimes problems just won't go away so 'heads must roll' and ruthless managers will have taken the trouble to identify a scapegoat. Lining up several fall guys offers choice and protects against the appearance of picking on any one individual; it is best to cast the net wide. In one case I heard of, a junior consultant was 'used' to eliminate a senior consultant who objected to part of the service being closed. She helped the managers build a case against her senior colleague by providing them with a log of late attendances to clinics, accounts of allegedly being uncontactable when on call and examples of lack of support for trainees, midwives and ancillary staff. The senior consultant was 'encouraged' to take early retirement. Adverse clinical outcomes followed, most probably due to insufficiently experienced staff in charge, but these root causes were overlooked. Instead, the management team concluded that the junior consultant was a 'disruptive influence' and that she was 'underperforming'. Her case was referred to the GMC. In her naivety she had expected them to support her in her hour of need, but she had miscalculated. She was just there to make sure they could oust her senior colleague without any flies landing on them.

3. Micromanagement

Ensuring every directive set out by healthcare commissioners or healthcare regulators is implemented requires a limitless number of meetings. Attendance is driven by the fear of being left out or usurped. Goals change frequently and priorities are often conflicting. Issuing overcomplicated instructions or redirecting actions to achieve short-term goals is commonplace. Few meaningful decisions are made but many actions are generated – circulating the agenda or minutes, emailing the team with updates, filling in spreadsheets, drafting or redrafting reports, organising a satellite meeting for further discussion on a particular issue. If frontline staff use meetings as a platform to raise concerns, these are often overlooked, unless addressing them fits a management directive or target. This is how real problems in service delivery become submerged in the mass of trivial action points.

Meetings to discuss frontline workforce shortages, the single greatest threat to the service, are comical. One anecdote concerns a labour ward shift during the bleakest weeks of the Covid-19 pandemic. A very experienced labour ward coordinator was in charge assisted only by a consultant and a foundation year trainee. Two specialist registrars due to work that shift had been deployed to the intensive care unit. Half the midwives were absent due to Covid infection or exposure to Covid, so only three were present, including a supposedly supernumerary student midwife. Caesarean sections were conducted with no assistants. For several hours women laboured unattended without relatives present due to the pandemic. The student midwife was left in charge of a mother contracting prematurely with twins. One woman delivered in the observation bay while waiting for a room to be deep cleaned following the discharge of a Covid-positive mother. There was no time to be stressed, just jobs to be done. Later that day the labour ward coordinator received an email from her line manager stating how disappointing it was that she did not log on to that morning's Covid crisis Zoom meeting to discuss the roll-out of the new Covid care pathways due to come into force the following week. She calculated that there were 17 people at that meeting, eight of them midwives by training. None of them thought it appropriate to walk over to the labour ward, put on some personal protective equipment (PPE) and lend a hand.

4. Obsessive pursuit of targets

Meeting targets has become a central tenet of how NHS services are judged, despite little evidence they improve patient outcomes. There are two main reasons for this disconnect. First, most are moving targets so when audit data shows the service has fallen short, targets are simply redefined, changed or replaced. This is how the six-week wait became the eight-week wait for elective surgery and why some maternity units variably define major obstetric haemorrhage as anything between >2 litres or >1 litre, thus keeping the prevalence the same. 'Creative' use of data is particularly common in relation to labour ward acuity scores, a crude measure of the patient-to-staff ratio, measured at regular intervals throughout the day. Among frontline workers, it is common knowledge that denominator data is often fiddled, for example by 'removing' early labourers or women awaiting assessment in triage, to ensure that frontline staffing levels appear better than they are.

Second, targets change behaviour in ways that do not necessarily result in better care or improve outcomes. The best example is the four-hour A&E waiting time target, which simply required a patient to be 'assessed' or 'moved' from A&E without any requirement to undertake investigations or therapeutic interventions. As anyone who has attended A&E can attest, this target can be met by moving a patient from one area to another within the four-hour window, then moving them on again within the next four-hour window. In maternity, there is plenty of evidence that chasing targets can be harmful. The most shameful example of this was the fixation with the national caesarean section rate which dominated practice for two decades.

This is such an important point that it is worth discussing the background to the caesarean section rate target in some detail. In 1985, the WHO convened a meeting of international obstetric experts to discuss the increasing medicalisation of childbirth, focusing in particular on the rising caesarean section rates worldwide. They concluded that 'there was no justification for any region to have a caesarean section rate higher than 10–15 per cent' (WHO 1985) because above this rate there was no statistically significant improvement in maternal or infant *mortality*. There was no mention of the enormous *morbidity* associated with futile or difficult labours, and absolutely no suggestion that mothers' preferences should be considered. Healthcare commissioners seized upon this target, agreeing unanimously that the UK caesarean rate was 'too high' and that this was costing the NHS 'too much' – meaningless terms that seemed not to consider the costs and consequences of not offering caesarean section to mothers who needed (or indeed wanted) this mode of delivery. The 15 per cent caesarean section target was music to the ears of the National Childbirth Trust (NCT), a national pregnancy and childbirth charity, which set up the Maternity Care Working Party in 1999, a group that included members of the RCM and RCOG. Their efforts culminated in the publication of the 'Normal Birth Consensus' (Maternity Care Working Party 2007) and the widespread rollout of the 2010 NICE toolkit aimed at achieving the 15 per cent target, which was well supported by midwives (Baldwin et al 2010).

Subsequent maternity care strategies were built around an almost evangelical belief that this was the only correct path to follow (Romano & Lothian 2008; National Maternity Review 2016; Black et al 2016), but chasing this target promoted some of the worst practices seen on NHS labour wards. Futile inductions of labour, prolonged use of oxytocin to augment labour, collective inertia in response to concerns in fetal heart rate monitoring, promoting excessively prolonged second stages of labour and risky if not damaging attempts at operative vaginal delivery became commonplace. Maternity units with low caesarean section rates were rewarded with extra funding under the payment by results (PbR) scheme (Department of Health 2013). The maternity unit at Shrewsbury and Telford Hospital NHS Trust became the exemplar of perfect maternity care when its leaders proudly reported a caesarean section rate of 16.3 per cent in 2013–14, compared with the national average of 26.2 per cent at the time (Ockenden 2022). Decisions to perform caesarean deliveries were challenged constantly by service organisers. Units thought to have 'too high' a caesarean section rate were regularly ordered by commissioners to perform a 'deep dive' into their clinicians' decision-making and asked to justify their intervention rates or send their non-compliant obstetricians for 're-training'. These were often senior clinicians who did not yield to the prevailing pressures and resolutely refused to embrace reckless practices. These objectors were ritually mocked for not being brave enough to foist prolonged labours upon exhausted mothers or embark upon difficult or damaging operative vaginal deliveries.

In one anecdote, a senior obstetrician was criticised for performing a caesarean delivery in a multiparous woman with meconium-stained liquor and a pathological CTG recording. 'What were you thinking?' the head of midwifery barked at the data review meeting. 'I was trying to save the baby from brain damage,' came the plucky retort, which invited the deplorable response, 'Well, that's not my problem – funding for that comes from the paediatric budget.'

Management teams in some trusts wrote letters to women advising them that they were not able to support requests for caesarean section without a clear medical indication and advised them to book elsewhere if they still 'insisted' on this mode of delivery. NHS maternity services were effectively turning their backs on women whose choices were not aligned with national targets, while at the very same time championing women's right to choose. The stench of hypocrisy was unbearable. Frontliners who dared to challenge the lunacy of it all were silenced: they had to get with the plan or get out. Job descriptions for senior positions in midwifery invariably mentioned a commitment to 'championing natural birth' among the essential attributes. Most bizarrely of all, even for obstetricians, whose job it is to offer and perform caesarean sections, consultant interviews in some trusts required prospective candidates to give a short presentation on what actions they would implement to lower the caesarean section rate should they be appointed.

Some units offered women who were fearful of vaginal birth psychiatric review, sending out the clear message that only 'mad' women choose caesarean birth. Women who had had caesarean deliveries previously posed a particular problem and money was thrown at the nationwide establishment of so-called 'birth options' or 'birth choices' clinics. This was essentially a tick-box exercise in which carefully chosen members of staff understated the risks of attempting vaginal birth after caesarean (VBAC) while disproportionately promoting the benefits. The fact that failure to offer caesarean delivery in a timely and proactive way can result in a range of disabilities in an infant and, in the most severe cases, condemn the family to a lifetime of round-the-clock care was disregarded. At the height of this phase, many frontline staff suffered from psychological stress and insomnia. My colleagues regularly described waking up in the middle of the night startled and sweating with terror at the thought of what was happening on the nation's labour wards. Some left the profession or took early retirement.

Despite the Morecambe Bay Report of 2015 specifically highlighting the perils of promoting 'vaginal birth at all costs', it was only in March 2022, after other independent national inquires described the tragic consequences of this policy, that the head of the RCM finally issued a half-hearted apology for the part this organisation played in creating an ideological culture around promoting 'natural birth' but caveated this with the accusation that some frontline midwives had 'misinter-preted' the directives. Mothers and babies paid the price; frontline staff got the blame. The target, like most, was never met.

5. Sycophantic interactions with healthcare commissioners and regulators

Successful meetings with healthcare commissioners are dependent upon slick PowerPoint presentations that focus on funding and demonstrate action in response to concerns. Meetings provide a platform for managers to 'pitch' their services in a series of embarrassing marketing rituals in which they describe a service that no frontliner or service user would recognise.

The day of the CQC inspection is the highlight of the management calendar and requires dusting down the old uniform worn at the last inspection. This exciting event represents the culmination of months of poring over data, addressing every target set following the previous inspection, sending out an infinite number of emails, ticking hundreds if not thousands of boxes, laminating notices on pinboards, rewriting fire safety protocols and coaching shop floor staff on what to say if questioned by inspectors. A last-minute splurge of funds on unblocking drains, pest control, cleaning the premises and improved signage should do the trick. How could the inspectors fail to award a better rating this time?

During one such inspection, the head of midwifery was showing inspectors around the ward. She marched up to us and confidently introduced me as Dr X, and I introduced the four other members of the team. There was some polite head nodding, but the conversation was dominated by the head of midwifery who continually praised me by name for the enormous contribution I had made to the unit, also stating how proud she was of 'her' team and how happy everyone was to work at the trust. Once they moved on, my colleague chuckled, 'That's funny, you don't even look like Dr X.' But why would the head of midwifery know who I was? She had been there for barely two years; two months later she was gone. Apart from the obvious comedic value to such interactions, they act as a constant reminder that the service is being organised by those who know nothing about service delivery.

6. Ignorance of basic operational matters

Independent national maternity inquiries regularly mention lack of visibility of managers in clinical areas and note limited interactions between managers and frontline staff or service users. This is because many view frontline staff as nameless subordinates and patients' problems as a matter for someone else to deal with. For example, managers rarely tell a mother directly that her elective caesarean section has been cancelled or her induction of labour postponed. These 'dirty jobs' are left to frontline staff.

Managers often have limited knowledge of the tools frontline workers need to do their job. The mass of red tape that surrounds NHS procurement policies is an area of particular concern, and the public got wind of this during the Covid pandemic in relation to PPE. In some maternity units, it took months for management committees to sanction the use of PPE for obstetric sonographers, who, everyone else seemed to agree, could not possibly do their jobs in a socially distanced way. Despite national and international recommendations to prioritise these members of frontline staff, by the time adequate supplies were issued, so many were off work due to infection or exposure to infection that pregnant women often missed out on time-sensitive scans.

Availability of equipment is largely determined by cost but often these are false economies, like the use of cheaper and ill-fitting gloves that tear frequently, requiring several glove changes per procedure. In one anecdote, a manager ordered 2,000 units of a piece of equipment not used in obstetrics 'by mistake', and staff were instructed to 'use these up' before the correct ones could be ordered. 'To do what?' one obstetrician asked. She then suggested sending the unwanted equipment to the main theatre department where the general surgeons, who regularly used this equipment, could make use of it in return for some funds to purchase the correct equipment. This simple and obvious swap took over three months to achieve because each division within the trust had a team of managers who had to decide whose budget would be affected and to what extent before approving it.

While issues relating to staff management or procurement may not be immediately obvious to patients, it would be difficult for them not to recognise the problems with inefficient workflows, a direct result of lack of managerial presence or understanding of operational matters. Many different services operate within maternity – outpatient clinics, outreach clinics, laboratories, ultrasound scanning rooms, maternity daycare, birthing units, labour wards, postnatal wards and so on. Some maternity units are part of a wider multi-speciality hospital, others stand-alone facilities. After delivery, some of the care is provided by community midwives and GPs. Occasionally, specialists in other fields need to be engaged. Complications might require transfer to a high dependency unit or even an intensive care unit. A preterm or poorly baby may need admission to a neonatal intensive care unit. Some mothers will need mental healthcare input from a mother and baby unit or involvement of social workers. And workload in one area inevitably impacts on another. For example, in 2015 the laudable aim of reducing the UK stillbirth rate by 50 per cent by the year 2025 was announced (DHSC 2015) and trusts were mandated to introduce several safety measures. Many managers signed up to these in principle without considering the practicalities, such as the 30 per cent increase in requests for obstetric ultrasound scans or the resultant 20 per cent uplift in inpatient admissions due to the increase in number of inductions of labour.

7. Crushing of dissent or objection

In my experience, if managers cannot achieve goals smoothly, they often default to the time-honoured practices of undermining 'protestors', bullying anyone who questions instructions, threatening staff with their livelihoods or withdrawal of certain services, horse-trading assets without consultation and blackmailing objectors. The countless examples of staff who have been suspended and referred for investigation to the NMC or GMC bear witness to these behaviours. 'Problem individuals' can be reprimanded for being a few minutes late for work, forgetting their name badge or wearing jewellery, whereas the same issues are blithely overlooked in those considered compliant. Once the non-conformer is identified, managers set about building a case against them because it is easier to bring about disciplinary action than undertake the onerous job of remedying the underlying causes of workplace conflict. Clinical incompetence is the easiest route to take but, if this proves difficult, there is always probity, prejudicial behaviour or impropriety. The next step is to isolate the individual by creating doubt in the minds of others. Rumour, gossip and corridor chats are helpful in achieving this, but nothing is committed in writing. Loyalty to the managerial cause offers a more peaceful existence, so many fellow frontline staff fall silent at this stage, not because they think their colleague is guilty but because they do not want to be goaded into a state of conflict which may backfire. Frontline staff know that self-censorship is intrinsically linked to survival. Realpolitik wins the day.

Despite the now mandatory processes in place to protect them (NHS England 2017a), the plight of whistleblowers in the NHS is a truly sad one and includes reputational damage, destruction of a hard-earned career, financial ruin, poor mental health, misuse of alcohol or other addictive behaviours, depression and even suicide (England 2020; Duffy 2019; Duffy 2021). When I was applying for my consultant post, a mentor explained the way this works. He described how a 'troublemaker' in his department was isolated and offered a diminished role. During the investigation, support for this doctor became lukewarm. Only my mentor had remained a stalwart supporter and, as I found out later, even went as far as attending the GMC tribunal in support of his colleague. The departmental silence was due to the so-called 'right to confidentiality while under investigation', which is tantamount to a non-disclosure agreement and mainly offers protection to the accusers because the doctor under investigation is unable to garner support in their defence. Like most GMC referrals the case was subsequently closed, and unlike most who are subjected to this process, this doctor went on to rebuild a successful career once vindicated. I asked my mentor whether his continued support had been ideological, perhaps a commitment to seeing justice being served. 'Oh no,' he said rather cheerfully. 'It is far simpler; it's just maths. It takes more than three years for the management to get rid of a doctor and I am retiring in two. I was the only one in the department who could afford to tell the truth without them coming after me too.'

An entire industry has grown up with the aim of restoring fractured relationships between frontline staff who have dared raise their heads above the parapet and their managers. There are toolkits and management training courses and, failing that, a wide choice of external agencies that can be engaged in conflict resolution (NHS

England 2017b). In theory, impartial facilitators encourage disputants to reveal their perspectives and feelings about the situation and enable the warring parties to find solutions. In practice, none of this is achieved, because the 'resolution event' is typically commissioned by the senior management team in collaboration with the trust's HR department once the large sums of taxpayers' money needed to fund this have been approved. Participants are told they must submit an account of their grievances without open discussion with colleagues prior to attending the resolution meeting. Interestingly, they cannot opt out of this supposedly 'voluntary' process and dismissal from the meeting is conditional upon the signing of a mediation agreement or similar. The HR representative, a manager, whose job it is to ensure numerous arcane processes are followed, usually chairs the events. The optics leave no doubt in the minds of any frontline worker as to where the balance of power lies. Hours, in some cases even days, go by and then the mediation agreement is signed never to be looked at again by either side. At the end of one mediation, a colleague overheard the mediator say to the HR representative, 'So which department are we doing next week?' Such is the demand for this service.

Many trusts have their go-to mediation company on speed dial, and mediators keep lining their pockets with taxpayers' money. Because the whole process is shrouded in secrecy, it is impossible to obtain data on just how much the NHS spends on dispute resolution, but the outcomes are always the same: a brief period of pretence at civility followed by a relapse into the same behavioural patterns as before. The chain is only broken when key protagonists move on to work elsewhere and as senior managers rarely stay in post for any length of time, frontline staff learn to just ride this out. Otherwise, there is often another mediation some months or years later and so the cycle continues. The most I have heard of anecdotally is four mediations involving the same individuals in about as many years. Rumour has it that mediations can cost between £5,000 and £30,000, not to mention the cost to patient care resulting from absent frontline staff. Many maternity units featured in independent national maternity inquiries have been through this process, a universally futile one because it fails to address the core issues giving rise to disharmony.

8. Lack of vision and strategy

Independent national inquiries into maternity care often describe leadership teams that lack vision and strategy. The vision should be obvious, namely the best possible clinical outcomes for mothers and babies. As such, every strategy should contribute to achieving this. But in the NHS, 'success' is not measured according to clinical outcomes but rather by the ability to deliver on directives set out by healthcare commissioners and healthcare regulators. Thus, reaching targets becomes the vision (because this translates into improved ratings), and implementing processes becomes the strategy. This has been the direction of travel since the 1990s, and the net result is a service organised according to managerial incentives rather than patient needs. And because tension and unrest are exhausting, managers surround themselves with like-minded people. Despite the assertion that fresh thinking and new ideas are welcome, NHS management teams are perfect examples of echo chambers. Time and time again, I have witnessed appointments of suitably obsequious individuals result in the creation of a progressive monoculture, only capable of propagating existing orthodoxies. Hardly the perfect breeding ground for the much-yearned-for improvements in the maternity service.

Conclusion

The past few decades have brought a shift in the balance of power in favour of management teams, who have shaped the maternity service with growing legitimacy and dominance. There has been a concomitant and progressive depletion, disempowerment and disengagement of frontline staff, who feel increasingly enslaved by a system in which their input is undervalued and disregarded in favour of operationally naïve individuals willing to pursue partisan priorities. Unsurprisingly, defections are common, with many frontline staff moving over to the winning team.

The fundamental problem is the confusion that has arisen by applying private sector management principles to healthcare services. In other organisations, managers are employed to enhance productivity and revenue, increase profit margins, invest in technology and innovation and encourage change with a view to expanding the business. Such organisations reward successful managers with bonuses or shares which encourage loyalty and longevity in post. Contrast this with the NHS, where managers work with limited resources within non-profitmaking organisations where contraction and centralisation of services are prioritised. Career progression within the fixed NHS salary scales mandates frequent moves to other NHS organisations resulting in a series of transient roles characterised by failure to address problems, lack of accountability, poor service development and no long-term vision, a situation one independent national maternity inquiry described as 'a leadership team in a constant state of churn and change' (Ockenden 2022).

I believe there are several steps that need to be taken in relation to service organisation. These include:

✦ making a clear distinction between clinical and non-clinical activity for all clinically trained staff on the NHS payroll so that the exact sums of taxpayers' money spent on management activity, both within and beyond trust level, can be determined
✦ being honest about the extent to which management directives shape the clinical service offered to service users
✦ analysing whether meeting management directives genuinely improves clinical outcomes
✦ establishing clear lines of accountability when standards fall short of expectation so as to guard against wrongful blame
✦ investigating the root causes of strained relationships between frontline staff and managers
✦ creating an environment in which service organisers are encouraged to prioritise service development over personal career development.

In the next chapter, I will return to the clinical arena and focus in more detail on how management-driven priorities have influenced care delivery with reference to maternity safety strategies.

5 Maternity care safety strategies – why do they fail?

Introduction

In the previous chapter, I discussed how NHS service organisers are required to measure 'quality' and 'efficiency' of healthcare services, address concerns regarding variation in standards of care nationwide and have systems in place that identify and deal with underperformance. In this chapter, I discuss how these priorities have shaped NHS maternity safety strategies.

Clinical governance

NHS safety strategies fall under the umbrella term of 'clinical governance' formally introduced as a new paradigm for teaching and practising clinical medicine in 1998 (Scally & Donaldson 1998). Clinical governance is 'a system through which NHS organisations are accountable for continuously improving the quality of services and safeguarding high standards of care by creating an environment in which excellence in clinical care will flourish'. Originally, it had several components, referred to as the 'seven pillars' – clinical effectiveness, audit, education and training, risk management, staff management, information management and patient and public involvement, but many more have been added over the years.

I remember when clinical governance was first discussed at a regional maternity meeting. There was widespread amusement in the audience because the so-called 'new ideas' being introduced had already been operational in UK maternity services for decades. One of the reasons the demise of NHS maternity services is quite so painful is that this speciality had been ahead of the game for so long. This is not intended to be self-congratulatory: there is little point basking in former glory if you have fallen from great heights. I say this because maternity is in many ways the canary in the coal mine for other medical disciplines. This once trailblazing speciality, an early adopter of all things new, has unwittingly become an example of how well-intentioned policies can lead us down a slippery slope towards potentially irreversible damage if they are implemented for the wrong reason and without scrutiny, or executed in the wrong way without rigorous intellectual debate about the potential consequences. The road to Hell is often paved with good intentions, and this will be clear when I describe the various components of clinical governance and consider the theoretical basis for their introduction and then contrast this with what has happened in practice.

Clinical effectiveness

There are two strands to clinical effectiveness. The first is establishing best practice using data from randomised controlled trials (RCTs); the second is using this information to standardise clinical care so that any treatment provided results in the best outcome for the patient. In 1993, the Cochrane Collaboration (cochrane.org), an independent global network of researchers, was established to collate and summarise evidence from multiple RCTs and the results of these meta-analyses are captured in guidelines and protocols issued by national organisations such as NICE. In the UK, all new medicines or procedures must be approved in this way. In the case of products and procedures still in the research phase, approval for use must be sought from the clinical ethics committees and administration requires written consent from participating volunteers. It sounds sensible in theory, but how does it play out on the shop floor?

Evidence-based practice

Many recommended medicines and procedures have been introduced on tenuous observational data rather than RCTs. Cost plays an important part in determining which are 'approved'. Let us take induction of labour as an example. The inexplicably popular 'cervical sweep' method is often used to kick-start labour. This requires verbal consent from the mother, a digital vaginal examination and the insertion of a finger into the cervical canal, which is 'swept' around between the fetal membranes and cervix to release local hormones that can prompt the onset of labour. In most cases, the procedure does not work except in those women who were going to labour in the next day or so anyway. National guidelines allow this to be performed on more than one occasion which, apart from being futile and uncomfortable for the mother, can also potentially introduce intrauterine infection. However, it is an inexpensive intervention and favoured by mothers who wish to avoid medical intervention. Because it does not work, the cervical sweep is usually followed up with one of several alternative methods of induction – tablets, gels, pessaries or balloon devices, all aimed at 'ripening' the cervix. Slow-release agents have become popular in recent years because they are cheaper and licensed for outpatient use: two factors which could result in cost savings. Unfortunately, in most cases where induction of labour is advised there are clinical concerns making outpatient use inappropriate. Also, the slow-release aspect means that in most cases at least 24 hours go past without much happening, and then the more expensive induction agents are required. Thus, the cost savings made by approving the cheaper drugs are rapidly offset by the extra costs associated with prolonged inpatient stay and unpredictable therapeutic response. This has prompted some pragmatic and well-informed women to ask for the 'induction medication that works'.

Evidence-based practice has always had its opponents (Greenhalgh et al 2014), and I have long been one of them because in obstetrics it has particular shortcomings. Comparing two different interventions or drugs for the treatment of a disease may give you different outcomes or cause the pathological process to run a different course and thus yield reasonable evidence that one is superior to the other. But because pregnancy is a physiological process and not a disease, comparing outcomes is trickier and, as I alluded to in Chapter 2, even if nothing is done the outcomes are more than likely going to be good. Let us look at the often-quoted RCT comparing intermittent auscultation (IA) of the fetal heart versus continuous electronic cardiotocograph (CTG) monitoring in labour. Both are supposed to provide reassurance that a fetus remains well during labour and pick up early signs of fetal distress. RCTs comparing the two have repeatedly shown that use of continuous CTG monitoring in low-risk pregnancies simply increases intervention rates such as operative vaginal deliveries or caesarean sections without necessarily avoiding poor neonatal outcomes such as hypoxic ischaemic encephalopathy, the leading cause of cerebral palsy (Alfirevic et al 2017). Many have taken this to mean that IA is not only just as safe as continuous CTG monitoring but has the added advantage of avoiding unnecessary intervention, so IA continues to be widely practised in low-risk labours throughout the UK. But in doing so they have missed the point completely. In IA, the fetus remains unmonitored for much of the time because national guidance mandates monitoring for one minute every 15 minutes in the first stage of labour (so the fetus is unmonitored for 90+ per cent of the time), and for one minute every five minutes, or for one minute after each contraction, in the second stage of labour (so unmonitored for about two thirds of the time) (NICE 2022). Because labour is a physiological process, a healthy, full-term fetus will more than likely be fine whether monitored or not. Thus, all the IA versus CTG trials have really proved is that continuous CTG increases intervention because if you look for a problem you are more likely to find it, and if you find it of course staff feel obliged to do something about it. In other words, use of continuous CTG monitoring is more likely to prompt proactive care, but with IA you will 'get away with' inaction despite the prolonged periods of no monitoring because the chances are the fetus was well anyway. To establish whether IA is truly 'safe' practice, the appropriate RCT would be IA versus no monitoring at all. Try getting that past a clinical ethics committee.

Clinical guidelines

Having, in theory, established what 'best practice' is, the second strand of clinical effectiveness requires this to be enshrined in clinical guidelines. The pocket-sized *vade mecum* of old I described in Chapter 3 has been replaced with ever-expanding electronic pages of definitions, advice and appendices available at the click of a mouse or tap of a mobile phone screen. These are updated regularly with the main aim of standardising practice. Today's trainee midwives and obstetricians can regurgitate the latest guidelines verbatim with the bland monotony they deserve, yet huge variations in practice are still seen throughout the country (Richmond & Sherwin 2021). Why has the plethora of clinical guidelines at our disposal not improved clinical outcomes? Well, there are several reasons for this:

1. Alteration

It is appropriate to change guidelines when new evidence comes to light, and there are nationally agreed timetables for updates after which 'old' guidelines are catalogued and filed away. These are occasionally useful when reporting on historical cases, but in theory they should be decommissioned. All too often, however, they remain in circulation. Additionally, trust clinical guidelines committees have the power to ratify trust-specific adaptations to national guidelines. While understandable and permissible, such alterations make a mockery of standardised care, and when poor outcomes occur it begs the question as to why the nationally agreed gold standard was not followed.

2. Duplication and proliferation

There are often a bewildering number of guidelines covering the same topics, with NICE guidelines, RCOG guidelines, regional, local and trust-specific guidelines often being referred to at the same time. Different hospitals within the same trust can sometimes use different guidelines, or two different guidelines can be used in parallel. The best example of this is in regard to intrapartum fetal heart rate monitoring, a problem perpetually noted in independent national maternity inquiries. Some units use NICE guidelines, others Federation of Gynaecology and Obstetrics (FIGO) guidelines, or physiological CTG interpretation, or the 'DR C BRAVADO' mnemonic from Advanced

Life Support in Obstetrics (ALSO). This is confusing and makes comparisons between units impossible.

3. Lack of clarity

Problems with clarity could be down to poor grammar and punctuation, or it could be that guidelines are left deliberately vague to allow clinicians some latitude in interpretation. Some are written specifically in response to a recent complaint or defensively following a litigation case. A seasoned guideline reader will be able to determine this. Sometimes the writing is so sloppy that the information provided is obviously contradictory. One trust, conscious of these problems, engaged a medicolegal solicitor to assist in redrafting guidelines and in her short time in post before the funding for this venture dried up, hardly a single page was returned without large chunks of text being highlighted for correction.

4. Unworkable in practice

Some guidelines are manifestly unworkable in practice, such as those related to consent for operative vaginal delivery (RCOG 2020) or caesarean section (RCOG 2022). These are utterly absurd insofar as they suggest frontline staff should reel off a list of horrific outcomes according to likelihood of occurrence with no mention of the individualised risks or potential benefits of intervention, and no obligation to inform the mother of the possible consequences of declining the procedure being offered.

5. Overshooting purpose

Our addiction to guidelines means their supposed purpose has been extended well beyond what is logical and reasonable. They have now replaced medical textbooks and other learning materials. For example, guidelines on the management of multiple pregnancy usually start with a definition of the word 'twins' or 'triplets' and then go on to discuss placental 'chorionicity' (the number of placentas) over several pages before one gets to the part that might assist in providing care to the mother and her babies.

In the past, guidelines were restricted to clinical matters, but now there are guidelines on every aspect of service provision, including how to conduct a handover between shifts, how to break bad news to a patient, how to deal with an aggressive relative and so on. Also 'clinical' guidelines now overlap with standard operating procedures in a bizarre, nonsensical mix of directives leaving frontline staff believing that no aspect of patient care can be provided without a formal set of instructions. Guidelines have not only replaced clinical knowledge and practical experience but also common sense.

6. Fundamental limitations

The biggest problem with guidelines, whether they are national, regional, local or indeed unit specific, is that they cannot possibly cover every clinical scenario. Neither can they capture the compulsion to deviate from standard practice, nor alter the threshold for intervention in the face of dual pathology. For example, the gestation at which induction of labour is recommended in a mother with gestational diabetes as well as hypertension may be different if she only had one or other of these conditions. Similarly, a borderline suspicious intrapartum CTG may prompt earlier delivery in a fetus known to be exposed to meconium-stained liquor, compared with the same CTG when the liquor is clear. Most importantly, when unusual presentations occur and lateral thinking is needed most, there is no guideline entitled 'Thinking Outside the Box'. The only way forward in these cases is through the seemingly lost art of taking a focused history, listening carefully to the answers, anecdotal recollection of similar cases and theoretical reasoning of potential differential diagnoses based on a sound knowledge of biological sciences and professional craftsmanship. Although these processes are scorned by the philosophies that underpin 'clinical effectiveness', and such notions are considered fanciful or even sacrilegious in our new age of formulaic care delivery, to my mind there is simply no substitute for thinking on your feet or even flying out on a wing and a prayer in a crisis.

7. Failure to protect both patients and frontline staff

A common misapprehension is that there is a correlation between following guidelines and achieving good outcomes, but simply following the recipe does not guarantee the perfect soufflé. Naïve clinicians also believe that following guidelines offers protection in the event of a poor outcome. This is also not true. A recurrent criticism raised in independent national inquiries and litigation cases is the lack of individualised care, but it should be perfectly obvious that care cannot possibly be both standardised and individualised at the same time. In practice, clinical guidelines often serve neither patients nor frontline staff, but they make for excellent reference sources when raising complaints or allegations of malpractice. And the more guidelines there are, the more ammunition is placed in the hands of the critics.

Audits

In theory, a clinical audit is conducted to assess whether clinical care is being delivered in accordance with guidelines: essentially a quality assurance process. Deviations and variations in practice are examined and underlying causes addressed to enhance compliance. The audit is then repeated to ensure matters have improved. This is called the audit cycle. As guidelines are changed, new auditable standards are set. Audits can be done on a large scale, such as the numerous national maternity audits that exist, or a much smaller departmental scale.

Yet again, UK maternity played a pioneering role. It was the first medical speciality to publish a national audit into maternal deaths, in 1952. These publications have changed names over the years from Confidential Inquiry into Maternal Deaths and Deaths in Infancy (CESDI) to Centre for Maternal and Child Inquiries (CMACE) and subsequently Mothers and Babies: Reducing Risk through Audits and Confidential Inquiries across the UK (MBRRACE-UK) in 2014, but their principal purpose remains unchanged. They are generally of a high standard and rely on reasonably robust data collected via national reporting systems to analyse all stillbirths, and maternal and neonatal deaths (npeu.ox.ac.uk). Since 2014, reports have also focused on severe maternal morbidities such as sepsis, cardiac disease or epilepsy. NHS maternity services have a unique legacy here; these are great achievements, and the tradition must be upheld.

Unfortunately, the same cannot be said of small-scale local clinical audits. These are largely meaningless because the wrong incentives come into play. Even if we are prepared to overlook the fact that local audits are judging care against one of several, not particularly useful, clinical guidelines as discussed previously, it is impossible to ignore that audit topics are chosen not according to pressing clinical concerns within the department but rather according to the criteria set out by the Clinical Negligence Scheme for Trusts (CNST). This organisation was established in 2001 to handle clinical negligence claims on behalf of member trusts in a process that was administered originally by the NHS Litigation Authority (NHS LA). To become members, trusts had to record activity, demonstrate engagement with the full gamut of maternity safety strategies and provide a record of claims (NHS LA 2001). The NHS LA, since renamed National Health Service Resolution (NHSR), assesses these data and levies financial contributions accordingly. Certain audits need to be completed to maintain membership, such as those related to CTG interpretation and management of obstetric haemorrhage. Collecting this type of compliance data is boring and tedious, so audits often include the minimum stipulated number of cases and clinical information is often inaccurate or incomplete.

Proof that the required audits were undertaken comes in the form of dull presentations at biannual trust maternity audit meetings. Topics change according to CNST requirements, so audit cycles may not be closed and improvements in care are not sustained. For example, in one trust that scored poorly for post-caesarean wound infection, negative pressure wound dressings were introduced for all obese women. There was indeed a reduction in wound infections but, once the target was achieved, the procurement team decided to cancel further orders of these expensive dressings. Within weeks, the wound infection rates started to rise again, but as this was no longer an auditable standard, no further action was taken. Unsurprisingly, attention and resources are lavished upon targets that are cheap to implement and likely to yield good audit results quickly, such as the UNICEF Baby Friendly Initiative for promoting breastfeeding where compliance with the target was assessed by way of ticking a mandatory field on the electronic discharge notification to confirm the mother had received advice and support with breastfeeding. In practice, this was often achieved by dropping off a leaflet at the foot of her bed. Unsurprisingly, the audit showed 100 per cent compliance.

Education and training

Education and training in maternity ensure staff engage in continuing professional development (CPD) and keep their practice up to date. Maintaining professional registration for midwives and obstetricians is conditional upon providing evidence of CPD activity at annual appraisals and future personal development plans often focus on achieving specialist skills, certification, diplomas or even degrees. Frontline midwives and obstetricians are fully on board with this as they invariably have a genuine interest in their field and recognise that a satisfying career goes hand in hand with lifelong learning. A uniquely rewarding aspect of clinical work is the opportunity to attend conferences, which are usually buzzing with fellow professionals who want to present their research, learn more and exchange views for the benefit of their patients.

In practice, education and training fall into two categories – mandatory/compulsory courses and self-directed:

Mandatory training

1. Trust-based training

Maintaining membership of CNST requires maternity units to reach compliance targets of 90 per cent for mandatory training. Every year, staff need to complete courses covering a wide range of general modules, such as fire hazards, first aid and handling of sensitive patient information, and speciality-specific modules such as fetal heart rate monitoring in labour.

It is worth focusing on the perennial problem of fetal heart rate monitoring in labour because failures in this area of clinical practice contribute to more than 75 per cent of adverse outcomes and play a key role in many cases of acute fetal brain injury. I have discussed IA already, but it is the correct interpretation of CTG recordings that has remained an enduring problem since its introduction in the 1970s. Over the past 30 years, attempts to address this problem have resulted in the introduction of endless classification systems devised by any number of organisations listed previously in this chapter.

In the 1990s, most maternity units introduced stickers in patient notes, which had various fields midwives had to fill in to help them objectify CTG recordings at regular intervals during labour. Outcomes remained unchanged, so some years later the extra action of a countersignature was introduced to ensure a 'second opinion' from someone not immersed in primary conduct of the case, which sounded good in theory but again did not improve outcomes in practice. The move away from paper to electronic CTG recordings by the end of the 2000s meant the introduction of electronic signatures and countersignatures on drop-down screens and alarms to prompt timely reviews, but still no improvement in outcomes. In 2015, the RCOG recommended full-scale adoption of 'fresh ears' for IA and 'fresh eyes' for CTG interpretation, which was essentially a more formalised version of the previous systems (RCOG 2015). This approach required double-checking at hourly intervals, although why it was considered that this version of the 'second opinion' system might work where the others had not was unclear. And with most units struggling to provide enough midwives for basic care, the luxury of a second midwife to nip in and out of the room so frequently seemed rather fanciful. As expected, outcomes remained unchanged. Moreover, while earlier independent national maternity inquiries *did* find staff to be lacking in CTG training, recent inquiries have reported poor outcomes in units where compliance with CTG training was excellent. So why is it that despite a multitude of increasingly complex toolkits and categorisation systems, a plethora of interactive online training courses, weekly CTG meetings and robust compliance data, there has been no reduction in birth asphyxia, hypoxic ischaemic encephalopathy and cerebral palsy?

Well, CTG interpretation will remain an eternal problem for the very simple reason that the test itself is severely limited. Training focuses on classification based on certain features and even if this was determined correctly every single time, for example by applying artificial intelligence, the improvements we long for would not occur because while a plum normal recording in a term fetus might be reassuring, anything else correlates poorly with clinical outcome due to the vast overlap between physiological and pathological features. In other words, unless grossly 'abnormal', a 'concerning' or 'suspicious' CTG may well represent a normal fetal response to the physiological process of birth in many, but not all, cases.

Appropriate use of this very crude screening tool requires the carer to understand its limitations and in most cases treat the data it provides as a small and unreliable part of a much wider clinical story. An experienced midwife or obstetrician will do a full physical assessment of the mother first and then pass a cursory glance at the CTG before formulating a management plan. A less experienced one will base clinical management of the labour predominantly on the CTG recording. The advent of central monitoring stations in which the fetal heart rate recordings of several labouring mothers are simultaneously displayed on a big screen at the nursing station is, I fear, only going to make things worse because the less time a midwife spends in the room of a labouring women, the less information about the overall clinical situation is gleaned and therefore the more flawed the clinical decision making. How a mother moves or breathes matters. What she says to her attendants matters. Her facial expression needs to be observed carefully with each contraction. All this is part of a comprehensive assessment, vital aspects of care that cannot be distilled into a guideline, captured in a table or on a sticky label, or taught in an interactive online session or a simulation scenario. Only sustained exposure to real-world intrapartum care, providing face-to-face care, working alongside experienced senior frontline staff, palpating the maternal abdomen over the entire duration of a series of contractions, and being encouraged to think freely and logically about the maternal and fetal condition in each individual case, can do this. The only reason CTG monitoring is still used at all is that no one has found anything better. It does not tell us very much at all and when we convince ourselves that it does, we get into trouble. Time and time again.

2. Skills and drills training

Other acute responders, such as the police, firefighters and armed forces, do simulation training and safety drills, so frontline maternity staff should be no different. In recent years, the number of these interactive training programmes seems to have grown exponentially – ALSO (Advanced Life Support in Obstetrics), MuSiC (Multidisciplinary Simulation Training in Obstetrics), SOS (Strategic Obstetric Simulation), PROMPT (PRactical Obstetric Multi-Professional

Training), ECO (Emergencies in Clinical Obstetrics), ROBuST (RCOG Operative Birth Simulation Training), EaSi (e-learning and simulation for instrumental delivery) and so on. Some require annual attendance, others every two to three years, and as usual with 90 per cent attendance targets.

In my experience, frontline staff are generally supportive of this type of training, but there are several aspects that do not find favour with them. First, the regular automated emails stating, 'You have been identified as non-compliant with training – contact the training office to book your place on a course. Please note compliance data is due to be submitted by the end of the month.' Second, there is the 'teaching your granny how to suck eggs' aspect because course facilitators are often young individuals who have chosen to pursue a career in teaching and training which exempts them from clinical work (at least in part and especially out of hours as teaching takes place during the daytime). Third, many staff feel self-conscious jumping around and wrestling with rubber mannequins shouting like banshees as the training scenarios descend into a farcical display of amateur dramatics. Fourth, there is scant evidence of sustained improvement in clinical outcomes as a result of such training, save for studies conducted in trial centres, nationally and internationally, which report favourable data generally unable to be replicated elsewhere. Last, and most importantly, these training programmes unintentionally promote reactive rather than proactive care because they fail to emphasise what should be the most important safety strategy of all, which is taking avertable action. The best crisis is one that is avoided in the first place, and bizarrely, this message is never prioritised.

3. Human factors training

Human factors training was introduced in the mid-2010s, and UK maternity services now require annual updates with, yes you guessed, a 90 per cent compliance target. Unlike previous simulation training programmes, it focuses on the contribution made by ergonomic or cognitive factors and interpersonal relationships to clinical risk rather than the acquisition of practical skills needed to get you out of a pickle. A wave of local and regional courses has come our way as many jump onto this bandwagon and try to do it bigger, better, brighter and bolder. There are a host of catchphrases and acronyms – DuPont's Dirty Dozen, SHEEP (systems, human interaction, environment, equipment, personal), PACE (probe, alert, challenge, emergency), CUS (concerned, uncomfortable, safety issue) and so on. Training is based on the aviation model of safe practice and participants are taught an inexhaustible number of mnemonics that will supposedly help them recognise and respond appropriately in settings where there is increased risk to patients.

This obsession with applying to healthcare the principles of safety-related behaviour in the aviation industry has been with us for some time, not least in clinical risk management, covered later in this chapter. However, the enviable safety record in the aviation industry has never been replicated in healthcare and fairly basic scrutiny will quickly reveal several reasons why I believe safety principles from aviation are not transferable to healthcare:

✦ If you are unfortunate enough to be involved in a mid-flight aviation accident, the chances are you will not survive, whereas in an adverse clinical outcome you or your baby will more than likely survive, but one or both of you may be left seriously damaged: the old mortality versus morbidity conundrum. Negative outcomes are much more wide ranging in clinical care.

✦ In the aviation industry, if there are not enough staff to check you in or manage the aircraft, as happened in summer 2022 after the Covid pandemic, your flight will simply be cancelled. If you go into labour on a day when there are not enough frontline midwives (30–50 per cent of shifts), cancellation is not an option, but you will be short-changed as staff are forced to spread themselves thin.

✦ During a flight, the pilot and co-pilot are charged solely with getting you to your destination safely. Apart from a quick hello and goodbye when you enter and exit the aircraft, they do not have to chat to you, ask you how you think they should fly the plane, consider any preferences you have or deviate from their usual practice because you ask them to. Midwives and obstetricians are expected to know their patients and interact with them compassionately and kindly and accommodate their requests wherever possible. These acts of benevolence may result in protocols, safety standards or safeguarding procedures being breached, bypassed or overlooked. In the aviation sector no such accommodations are permitted; professionals focus purely on safety.

✦ If the onboard equipment does not work or the safety check is incomplete the pilot will not take off, yet midwives and obstetricians are expected to make do with whatever equipment and tools are available to them. Anyone who has ever opened a delivery pack to find a piece of equipment missing or started a caesarean section without a valid group and save sample (blood test sent to the laboratory to assist the timely crossmatching of donated blood in case blood transfusion is needed) will be familiar with this. The 'it will probably be fine' way of working so accepted in clinical practice is utterly unacceptable in the aviation industry.

✦ The cockpit is a safe space where the pilot and co-pilot can discuss and plan their actions without background noise and distraction. Contrast that with an ultrasound scan appointment where are noisy toddler has been brought in to 'see' its sibling, or family members who take videos of the birth, or the birth partner who takes over from the midwife and instructs the mother how to push. There is often a running commentary from relatives, TV or music playing loudly in the background, chatting on telephones, and the door flinging open and shut as people come and go. Frontline staff are expected to remain focused despite these distractions.

✦ In the aeroplane, the flight deck crew are expected to escort disruptive, rude or inebriated clients off the plane before take-off, or limit the amount of alcohol served to them during the flight if their demands are considered excessive. Passengers are expected to comply with instructions to wear safety belts and return to their seats at critical times during the flight. NHS staff are expected to work with whomsoever comes their way, without the right to impose any limits on antisocial, off-putting or abusive behaviours. Frontline staff are expected to safeguard patient dignity and confidentiality at all times, yet feel unable to object when they feel uncomfortable, undermined or threatened.

✦ Being a passenger in an aircraft is conditional upon the purchase of an airline ticket and as such may be regarded as exclusive and transactional. NHS healthcare is freely available to everyone and accessing it can be accompanied by a sense of entitlement. Thus, how a service is accessed can shape human behaviours and expectations.

If we adopted the same approach as the aviation industry, the healthcare service would grind to a halt. Our service is imperfect due to the fluid nature of human interactions, so comparison with a highly automated, robotic and entirely safety-focused service devoid of such exchanges is pointless (Kapur et al 2015).

Self-directed training

Self-directed training is a term used to describe any educational activity not necessarily required by the trust and these often have to be self-funded. While opportunities in healthcare management training are plentiful as outlined in Chapter 4, far fewer options exist for those who wish to achieve skills in patient-facing roles. Independent national maternity inquiries and RCM surveys frequently highlight this lack of support in clinical career development as a contributory factor to high staff turnover and attrition, a very real and frustrating problem for ambitious and talented frontline staff. Unfortunately, anything without a compliance target attached to it is simply not a priority.

Maternity risk management

In theory, maternity risk management aims to minimise risk to pregnant mothers and babies by analysing adverse outcomes or near misses so that 'the Service' can employ risk mitigation measures and prevent recurrence by 'learning from mistakes'. The process was originally adapted from existing risk analysis tools used in the airline industry. As ever, maternity was an early adopter and over the decades this process has become ever more complex. Investigations are supposed to be thorough and rigorously debated, the final report is sent to the healthcare commissioners, the findings are shared with staff and learning points are actioned. In recent years, to counter allegations of lack of transparency, concealment or collusion raised by independent national maternity inquiries, reports are also shared with service users who are invited to participate fully in the process.

Unfortunately, maternity risk management has not improved care. We know this because the same problems crop up again and again. More distressingly, this process has been instrumental in causing division and disharmony in the workplace and is widely regarded to be the main contributor to what independent national inquiries refer to as the 'blame culture' in many UK maternity units. From beginning to end, I believe this process is deeply flawed, open to abuse and frequently used for leveraging ill-considered gains. Let me describe it in more detail.

As mentioned previously, NHS trusts are required to report the most serious adverse outcomes such as mortality via national reporting systems, but for most other cases local reporting systems will suffice. The first step is notifying the clinical incident team that an adverse event has occurred which is, laughably, a voluntary process and involves submitting information via a trust IT reporting system or emailing a risk manager. Some staff report incidents frequently; others hardly ever. This information is then passed on to the maternity risk management panel, a group comprised of senior maternity managers, their deputies and a few clinicians. A report summarising the salient points is generated within a few days or weeks, but this initial assessment is sometimes patchy and often skims over the surface. There is ample opportunity for members of the maternity risk management panel to either overlook or highlight specific aspects of the incident according to a desired narrative. For example, a myriad of minor if not irrelevant points can be emphasised if the adverse event occurred in a unit earmarked for closure because of the need to provide evidence of underperformance. Similarly, inconsequential misdemeanours by unpopular staff can be embellished to help build a case against them. Serious problems may be swept under the rug if revealing them risks making a favoured individual look vulnerable, falling short on compliance targets or threatening a good service rating. These glaring inadequacies and flagrant abuses of the maternity risk management system are well documented in most independent national inquiries (Smith & Dixon 2007; Kirkup 2015; Ockendon 2020 and 2022).

Next, harm to patients is graded using words such as 'negligible', 'minor', 'moderate', 'severe', 'catastrophic' or a colour-coded system – green, amber or red. Grading systems are subjective so can result in what independent national maternity inquiries have referred to as 'inappropriate downgrading of incidents'. Attempts are then made to determine contributory factors but interestingly, insufficient staffing, which I would wager contributes to almost every adverse event, is usually placed in the 'minor contribution' category because it is presumed to cause delays in care delivery rather than frank harm. I suspect it would be the view of most frontline staff that this finding should deserve at least a 'moderate' if not a 'major' rating. The incident is then graded according to how likely it is to happen again, which is absurd because every frontline member of staff knows the correct answer to that question is 100 per cent, but this is rarely the box ticked. The most serious incidents used to be called 'never events', for example a retained surgical swab, and the target for recurrence is 0 per cent, but of course this is just pie in the sky.

For complex cases, a 30–60-day timeline to provide a report is allowed and the maternity risk management panel appoints one or more internal lead investigators who are expected to interview staff involved, collate statements, summarise the findings and identify areas of concern. All of this must be done while still maintaining the compulsory 'blame free' mantra. The investigator(s) writes a report according to a set template and submits this to the maternity risk management team. After many weeks or even months of toing and froing between various people's email inboxes, the case is finally presented at a risk review meeting, typically to a panel comprised of people with titles containing the word 'head', 'risk', 'lead' or 'safety', many of whom have nothing to do with the maternity service. Apart from all being on the same panel, these individuals usually share other things in common notably their meagre patient-facing commitments, negligible out-of-hours clinical responsibilities and non-existent first-hand experience of managing cases like the one being presented to them. This may seem bizarre until I explain that they are not there to understand the workings of the maternity unit or its problems. No, their job is, first, to generate a list of 'recommendations' or 'action points' and, second, to ensure the report is suitable for presentation to healthcare commissioners, healthcare regulators and service users.

This can be a tricky business. Recommendations and action points need to be credible enough to give the appearance of taking problems seriously, but not so pointed as to reveal irreparable deficiencies in the service. Healthcare commissioners and healthcare regulators are more likely to forgive one-off correctable blips rather than profound, long-standing and therefore potentially unrecoverable failings. As for the mother and her relatives, in my experience they are rarely placated by these reports and often exercise their right to reject the findings, request further clarification or suggest additional remedial actions. The final version of the report, which has been amended to reflect input from all parties, is often unrecognisable to the investigator(s) tasked with writing it in the first place, despite the fact that it still bears their name(s) on the front page. The completed process can take anything between several months to more than a year.

Ultimately, the list of action points almost always includes updating, altering or writing more guidelines, implementing another audit, changing prescribing policies or organising further training for frontline staff. Emails to frontline staff advising them of these matters follow. 'Learning points' are circulated via departmental newsletters, and yet more laminated safety notices are displayed wherever there is an inch of free wall space.

A recurrent theme raised during educational supervision meetings and appraisals is the treatment of frontline staff involved in adverse incidents who feel they were misrepresented or wish to appeal. Typically, they will be gently reminded, assuming they have not worked it out for themselves, that the maternity risk management panel is comprised of individuals who are perfectly positioned to 'shape' their career. Any suggestion that remedial actions are reactionary, disproportionate or biased is discouraged.

The Healthcare Safety Investigation Branch (HSIB, hsib.org.uk) later renamed the Maternity and Newborn Safety Investigations (MNSI, mnsi.org.uk) in 2023 is an investigatory body that was established in part to address the widespread recognition that NHS maternity risk management was used as a tool for bullying frontline staff (UK Parliament 2021). HSIB/MNSI investigation teams have the advantage of being unknown to the frontline staff they are investigating so are considered the more acceptable face of risk management. However, in practice they are simply a remote, online and dialled-down version of the local maternity risk management team.

Their panels often include ex-clinicians long retired from frontline duty, 'clinical' managers, patient advocates and a whole host of lay representatives and despite being nominally 'independent' they report to the CQC, which in turn reports to the DHSC. Frontline workers may feel less threatened by members of this panel, but in truth, the fact that the investigations are conducted by a group of semi-retirees attending a mid-morning meeting in an air-conditioned room, or logging onto an online meeting from the comfort of their home during a weekday and chatting about a sad case over a cup of tea and some biscuits before casting their verdict, is manifestly unjust, even if panel members are not in a position of direct power over those being judged. Like local trust-based maternity risk management reports, HSIB/MSNI reports are nowadays written largely for the benefit of service users and outline every medical term in layperson's detail to assist understanding. Despite nearly a decade's worth of national data being available to this organisation, there is no evidence of improvements in maternity outcomes and many, myself included, have concluded that this is just another expensive, taxpayer-funded, failed experiment.

Staff management

A safe maternity service needs intelligent workforce planning and the ability to engage and empower frontline staff so that the right number of workers with the right skill sets are available when and where needed. Anyone who is underperforming for any reason needs to be identified and helped to improve or adapt their working practice, within a discreet and supportive environment. Turning an underperforming or struggling member of frontline staff into a functioning employee requires appropriate and timely action by service organisers.

I discussed the staffing crisis in previous chapters and while adequate numbers are clearly a problem, so is skill mix. Not all midwives are equivalent, even if they are on the same pay scale. For example, there is no point deploying a high dependency unit midwife trained to monitor a patient with severe pre-eclampsia to the postnatal ward where the pressing concerns relate to supporting mothers with lactation. Similarly, a midwife who mainly works in a birth centre is not the best person to support the elective caesarean section list. And a midwife recently returned to work after a hip replacement might not yet be ready for a long shift on the labour ward but might function perfectly well in the antenatal clinic until she is fully recovered. Getting the best out of your existing staff and furthermore, being a good role model for students and trainees so they are encouraged to stay and contribute long term to the service, requires maternity managers to a) be present in clinical areas; b) know their staff well; and c) care that the clinical needs of patients are addressed appropriately. Unfortunately, 'staff management' is often reduced to chess-boarding an ever-decreasing number of names around an Excel spreadsheet to fill gaps, which results in the wrong combination of people in the wrong place doing jobs they are not well suited to do. Independent inquiries refer to this as 'dysfunctional teams'. Anyone who has ever tried to do a seating plan at a wedding knows it is not necessarily easy to get the right mix of people together, but even the least motivated would not leave it to chance alone.

The most unattractive aspect of staff management is managing underperformance. Managers must be sensitive, tactful and non-judgemental in determining the underlying causes and establishing whether they are temporary or permanent. Midwives and obstetricians, just like anyone else, can be the victims of ill health, stress, addictions, depression, anxiety, poor family relationships or, quite simply, burnout. Dissatisfaction with professional life is not unique to healthcare, but it is certainly made worse by a punitive system of managing underperformance. Threats of forcing an individual to work part time or work in another unit or join a team in which they are unlikely to thrive can compound the problem. Equally damaging is allowing underperformance to go unchallenged. In 2000, GP Dr Harold Shipman was found guilty of murdering 15 patients under his care over several decades, and closer to our own speciality neonatal nurse Beverley Allitt received 13 life sentences in 1991 for the murder of four infants, attempted murder of three others and grievous bodily harm to a further six, earning her the nickname 'The Angel of Death'. The public, quite rightly, expects only the highest standards of moral, ethical and professional behaviour from healthcare workers and, while these rotten apples do our profession no good whatsoever, our reputation is further damaged by reports that trust management teams often turn a blind eye to mounting evidence preferring instead to accept feeble explanations for a series of poor outcomes. This has prompted the publication of toolkits aimed at assisting managers to recognise and deal with underperformance (NHS Employers 2025) but the peripatetic nature of NHS managers makes me doubt they will succeed in weeding out the rot.

Information management

There are strict rules and regulations involved in the storage and sharing of clinical data and much of this is enshrined in the Data Protection Act and more recently the General Data Protection Regulation (GDPR). Once again, maternity services have form in this area. This was the first speciality to encourage handheld patient maternity records in the 1980s, although today most maternity units use an electronic version via a maternity care app or similar, which allows the mother to see her clinical data, blood results or scan reports, and manage her appointments. Should she require care elsewhere, she has remote access and control over her clinical data and is able to share it if needed. Overall, this works well, although it is important that those who are digitally excluded for any number of reasons, including poverty, poor educational background, language barriers, learning difficulties, poor mental health, visual impairment or limited access to handheld devices are not disadvantaged.

Patient information related to inpatient care sits within the problematic area of NHS IT systems and is not maternity specific, so I will not dwell on this save to say that the NHS has invested, or more accurately wasted, enormous sums of money on failed IT projects. In an attempt to meet the target of becoming paperless by 2018 several projects were instigated in the early 2000s, but by 2011 the NHS had clocked up a bill of £12 billion, and most projects were subsequently abandoned as they were beset by changing specifications, lack of technical support, complex software systems being run on archaic hardware and disputes as to what information was to be collected and how it was to be used. Any successful organisation will tell you that high-quality data means power: the power to assess demand for your service, staff it adequately, provide appropriate materials and equipment, engage in research and innovation, plan for unpredictable events or external shocks such as the Covid pandemic, anticipate future needs, invest resources wisely and base strategic planning on logical and robust grounds. Any service that is reliant on poor-quality data systems will not only miss out on these opportunities but may also leave itself vulnerable to cyberattacks such as those in 2023 and 2024 (Martin 2024).

Patient and public involvement

Public and patient involvement in NHS care has been operational informally for several decades but was formalised by way of the 'friends and family' test introduced in 2013 (NHS England 2013). In the future, I anticipate that service user input into maternity services will become the main focus of improvement strategies, work that is already under way through a network of charities and organisations, including National Maternity Voices, Birth Companions, Birthrights, Better Births, Maternity Action, Maternity Alliance, MumsAid, Association for Improvements in the Maternity Services, the Maternity Transformation Programme, National Maternity Voices and the Maternity Incentive Scheme.

As with most feedback systems, however, most users do not participate and many that do are driven by negative experiences. Nevertheless, having these feedback systems in place is required by healthcare regulators so they are supported by service organisers. In contrast, frontline staff are often indifferent to them. This is not because they do not care what users think as is often portrayed, but rather because patient feedback usually focuses on matters of expectation or 'experience' rather than safety. Much as one is likely to rate a restaurant by its atmosphere, friendliness of the servers or presentation and taste of the dishes rather than stating 'I am pleased that the restaurant kitchen meets the stipulated food hygiene standards'. The innumerable feedback forms I have read raise entirely legitimate concerns about clinic waiting times, delays in care, inflexible visiting times, limited menu options and so on. These are undoubtedly important issues, but many are not directly related to patient safety unless written retrospectively after a poor outcome, something politicians should remember when promoting reforms to maternity services based largely on consumer group feedback.

Other safety strategies

The 24/7 service and escalation

Following the Morecambe Bay inquiry, which suggested an association between poor perinatal outcomes and lack of senior staff availability, recommendations included moving to a 24/7 resident on-call obstetric consultant model. Maternity care by its very nature is a 24/7 service, but this directive mandated senior obstetricians to be present at all times making 'escalation' easier. This buzzword features in many adverse incident reports and medicolegal cases. At the time, this recommendation was also in line with the government's mandate to NHS England in 2016/17 to establish a seven-day NHS (DHSC 2015). NHS maternity managers throughout the country jumped onto this bandwagon as if their lives depended on it, but enforcing it turned out to be a very expensive mistake, which many units revoked soon after it became clear that it made no positive impact on patient care (Henderson et al 2017). It failed for the very simple reason that a consultant obstetrician on their own, without the presence of anaesthetists, neonatal staff, theatre staff, cleaners, porters, laboratory staff and, most crucially of all, midwives, is of no use whatsoever. Many spent the small hours of the morning sitting around on labour wards locked in a state of impotence but, worse still, the irrational gusto with which this policy was implemented resulted in the progressive disengagement, or premature retirement, of many senior obstetricians in their mid-to-late fifties who no longer wished to work the same shifts as their registrars, leaving some challenging situations to be dealt with by relatively inexperienced staff.

The requirement for junior staff to 'escalate' more and more cases has caused other problems because escalation means direct involvement of consultant obstetricians in many cases, which results in loss of oversight of the whole unit because the vital control and command role is compromised, similar to labour ward coordinators being pulled into direct caregiving previously described. Thus, working patterns today result, not infrequently, in situations where even senior staff cannot see the wood for the trees. Also, in obstetrics there is a tendency, maybe even an expectation, that once notified, seniors should then take over conduct of the case, causing deskilling of junior staff.

Fetal monitoring champions

Fetal monitoring champions are floor-walking midwives who assist frontline staff in CTG interpretation, provide 'fresh eyes' or 'fresh ears', conduct weekly training sessions and, naturally, ensure compliance with CTG training targets. The problem is that they don't walk the floor outside office hours and, in the words of one of my midwifery colleagues, 'the fetal monitoring champion was nothing more than a fetus herself'. In my view, this is just another example of inexperienced, non-clinically active staff telling the broken, dispirited frontline workforce how to do their jobs but not being there to help out when needed. Their presence simply ensures CTG training targets are met.

Safety huddles

Safety huddles were introduced in maternity units in 2019 as part of the NHS Improvement framework (NHS England 2019). The aim was to improve communication between staff working in different areas, a problem highlighted in independent national inquiries. In theory, representatives from all areas 'huddle' together at a meeting held online to discuss bed occupancy, staffing numbers, theatre scheduling, the need to transfer patients in or out from neighbouring units, concerns affecting workflows, supplies of equipment and so on. Many maternity units conduct these meetings daily, some even twice daily.

In practice, attendance by frontline staff is limited and patchy due to clinical commitments, so the meetings are dominated by non-clinically active staff and many of the policy decisions reflect this. In an anecdotal case of a mother carrying triplets who required preterm delivery, there was only one neonatal cot available at her intended place of delivery so the ingenious solution proposed was to transfer the mother to another unit which was 'only 25 miles away' where two cots were available, deliver her there and 'send the strongest baby back'. Scant thought was given to how the mother might care for three babies in two different locations, her recovery after caesarean section or the disruption to family life. In another case, the problem of not enough staff to complete discharge summaries was solved by sending a women home 'without the paperwork because we need the beds' and asking her or relatives to 'return later for her medication'.

Listening or 'open door' sessions

Listening or 'open door' sessions were originally suggested as a means of bridging the gap between a distant, aloof leadership and harassed, disgruntled frontline staff. The first step in this 'getting to know one another better' exercise is the issuing of personalised badges bearing names and designations – 'Hi! My name is BOB. I am HEAD OF MIDWIFERY' or 'Hi! My name is JACKIE. I am a MATERNITY CONSULTANT' or 'Hi! My name is ABDUL. I am a SONOGRAPHER'. Emails are sent out inviting frontline staff to come and chat to their interested and approachable manager because their 'door is always open' but only at times that suit them and never when they are working from home, or indeed after 5 pm, or at weekends. Some units call these 'Ask Me Anything' or 'Talk to X (insert manager's name)' sessions. In recognition that not everyone may have the time or feel comfortable attending such sessions, managers also arrange regular 'walkabouts' in clinical areas to demonstrate their availability, their ability to listen to the concerns of frontline staff, and their willingness to experience life at the coalface, albeit for a few seconds. Trusts often splash out on cakes or muffins, so they come bearing gifts. Sometimes a guest is invited to give a one-off talk on 'mental wellbeing' or similar. Hilariously, one event I witnessed involved a yoga teacher encouraging staff to sit on floor mats placed in the nursery of a postnatal ward and do gentle breathing exercises while babies cried and buzzers sounded in the background. A perfect way to relax and rejuvenate.

Conclusion

In this chapter, I have explained why maternity safety strategies have not improved clinical outcomes. I believe systems that genuinely protect patients from harm are contingent upon the following:

+ no longer misappropriating maternity safety strategies for managerial gain
+ moving away from target-driven commissioning processes and compliance-driven regulatory processes as they do not correlate with improved outcomes
+ ensuring safety directives to frontline staff are clear, concise and workable in practice
+ acknowledging that any safety strategy likely to produce improvements in clinical outcomes needs to be spearheaded by senior clinicians *in active practice*
+ being honest about the single greatest threat to the service, which is a lack of experienced frontline staff, and admitting that no safety strategy can compensate for this.

Safety strategies are supposed to ensure the best possible clinical outcomes for service users who arguably have the greatest vested interest in establishing a functional maternity service. In the next chapter, I will turn my attention to service users, the third stakeholder group.

Maternity service users – what do they want?

Introduction

I have left this important group until now because I wanted to describe the general maternity service landscape before exploring the role of service users. In recent decades, use of the word 'patient' has been discouraged in favour of 'customer' or 'client', a natural extension of the internal market philosophy. These words seem utterly absurd to older frontline staff for several reasons. First, one might be a regular 'client' at a restaurant or hairdresser, but few attend healthcare establishments through choice. Second, it assumes alternatives are available, but the NHS is a monopoly provider and data suggests only 0.4 per cent of women in England access private maternity care (National Audit Office 2013). Third, it suggests a relationship between client and service provider which is odd in a service where women hardly ever see the same member of staff twice. Last, words like 'client' and 'customer' are empowering and engender the belief that one can demand what one wants from the service, which risks raising expectations and offering false hope. Nevertheless, for the purposes of this chapter, I will use 'client'.

It is dispiriting to note that independent national inquiries increasingly conclude that clients and their relatives were not listened to, and their complaints and concerns were dismissed. In a service that is depleted of a stable and experienced frontline workforce and compensates for this by routinely employing clinical safety strategies that are unfit for purpose, it is not surprising that some clients feel they are being processed rather than cared for. Despite a concerted effort to move away from the 'midwife/obstetrician knows best' approach of the past, there continue to be reports of unacceptable behaviours (Care Opinion 2017; Murray 2024). In 2024, the CQC polled 20,000 clients and more reported negative experiences compared with previous years (CQC 2024). Poor access to out-of-hours care, lack of confidence in caregivers and inadequate communication were central themes. The Times Health Commission surveyed more than 1,000 mothers and one in four reported feeling that they or their babies were in danger, being 'fobbed off' or 'feeling powerless' to direct their care (Hayward 2023). In March 2023, the Parliamentary and Health Care Service Ombudsman reported that repeated failings in maternity care were putting mothers' and babies' lives at risk and questioned why lessons had not been learnt (Parliamentary and Health Care Service Ombudsman 2023). Anecdotes are often disturbing, with clients frequently identifying specific members of frontline staff they believe were responsible for their plight. It was that midwife who said 'x', that labour ward coordinator who did 'y', that registrar who failed to recognise 'z' or that on-call consultant who failed to attend. So serious are some of these allegations that after the publication of one independent national maternity inquiry, West Mercia Police set up Operation Lincoln (westmercia-pcc.gov.uk/operation-lincoln-support-for-victims), a specific team of officers tasked with investigating cases for potential criminal negligence to be filed against NHS trusts or individuals working within them.

NHS maternity services appear to be locked in a troubled state, all too often marred by customer dissatisfaction, anger, criticism and the quest for retribution. Thus far, I have discussed the changing roles, priorities and challenges service providers and organisers have faced, but the complex nature of what clients have come to expect from the maternity service and the reactions they have when the service falls short are worth exploring too.

Past and present challenges

Historically, the only thing a pregnant woman could hope for was that she and her baby would survive pregnancy and childbirth. This is still true in many parts of the world today. Women's access to contraception, the facility to avoid or treat sexually transmitted infection, the right to engage in sexual relationships without fear, violence or coercion and the ability to bear children safely and raise them in a supportive environment are all crucial components of a peaceful, stable and successful society (Humble 1995). In the UK, the NHS has been providing maternity care for several decades and, despite increasingly negative media accounts, many clients engage with the service in a positive way. It is considered fair as it is taxpayer funded and women feel entitled to use it because they have paid into it. They feel reassured that it is not a profit-driven service so there are no 'wrong incentives' as in other healthcare systems. Mothers who have delivered babies abroad speak of being charged extra for additional appointments or caesarean delivery; the NHS does not place limitations on the number of attendances. The modern maternity service is, at least in theory, in line with all the founding principles of the NHS. So admired is the NHS globally that it is often cited as a 'pull factor' for immigration to the UK, especially among young couples hoping to start a family. Media articles and TV documentaries have focused on 'health tourism' in UK maternity services. In recent years the popular press has reported that one in 20 women in NHS maternity wards are not entitled to NHS care, leaving many trusts in a desperate financial situation as it is impossible *not* to treat mothers and babies, and equally impossible to recuperate any money for the care provided (Adams 2020).

Over time, clients' expectations have changed. While their forebears would have been content simply to survive the process or be warmed by the fact that the service was free at the point of delivery, women in more recent generations have wanted more. Modern-day concerns focus on the lack of continuity of care and one-to-one care in labour, delays resulting in clinical deterioration, a confusing range of clinical care settings, inflexible scheduling of appointments and procedures, problems accessing specialist care, long clinic waiting times and patchy use of electronic records. Inequalities in maternity outcomes affecting clients who lack agency, social capital or educational privilege, while easily overlooked in previous generations, have become dominant themes. Poor communication, especially with mothers whose first language is not English, is often highlighted, a problem compounded by the fact that many frontline staff do not speak English as a first language so even officially recognised interpretation services do not always address all the issues perfectly. But there are other vulnerable groups too, including victims of domestic violence, drug addiction or poverty, travellers, the homeless, sex workers and those who have been trafficked. Many need perinatal mental health support, frequently referred to as the Cinderella service within the NHS, but a particular problem in maternity given findings of client surveys.

These concerns are legitimate and shared by frontline staff too, so calls to address them are justifiable. However, during my career, I have detected a gradual creep from reasonable expectation towards entitlement and unachievable ideals driven by what I consider to be damaging social narratives around pregnancy and childbirth. This has made the reality of providing maternity care that satisfies clients increasingly challenging, a task made more problematic by the fact that, unlike any other medical speciality, it is not just the 'client' frontline staff need to please. Having a baby is, it would seem, everyone's business and everyone has an opinion as to what is best. Advice based on anecdote, religious or cultural beliefs, superstition and old wives' tales abounds and is impossible to contradict. Everyone feels entitled to offer guidance on diet, lifestyle, vitamin supplements, general day-to-day activities, the birthing process and care of the newborn. Mothers-to-be are regularly asked intrusive questions by members of the public they barely know. Some even have their abdomens touched by strangers, which in any other context would, at the very least, be considered an invasion of one's personal space. These are not intended to be unkind acts – quite the opposite. They simply reflect the fact that everyone is emotionally invested in the outcome.

It is impossible to get excited about attending hospital for a chest X-ray or knee replacement, yet maternity clients, family members and friends attend antenatal clinic appointments full of joy, hope and expectation. They want to be reassured that all is well, get a 'photo' of the baby on scan or 'hear' the baby's heartbeat. In every other speciality, encounters with healthcare services are considered irritating events that must take place to restore health to what it was prior to the affliction. But pregnancy is different: it is a physiological process, it is 'natural', it is not a disease or an illness. And therein lies the problem. Pregnancy and childbirth today have been glamourised, romanticised and commercialised to the point that in people's minds pregnancy-related problems are consigned to history. Maternal death – surely a thing of the past? Stillbirth and infant death – surely only in the developing world? Media reports of harm are taken to be unfortunate one-offs, hyperbolic accounts of isolated bad outcomes, something that happens to someone else. And the social stigma that surrounds miscarriage, fetal loss, stillbirth and infant death does not help because it means that few are willing to talk about these matters. This contributes to a conspiracy of silence that surrounds many unsuccessful pregnancies. How has this mismatch between expectation and reality come about?

Information provided to maternity clients

In the past, women hoping to fall pregnant or in the early stages of pregnancy had limited sources of information, mainly mothers or aunts or perhaps an older sister who might have gone through the process more recently. These people were not professionals but likely to be supportive and well meaning. Later in the pregnancy, discussions with midwives would have provided more objective information. Midwives of old had the experience and confidence to, politely but firmly, disabuse mothers-to-be of any preconceived notions, but information was typically given on a need-to-know basis. Midwives had the upper hand. Women presented in labour, usually alone, not really knowing what to expect. Many felt their care was determined according to what their carers considered appropriate. They would certainly not have considered themselves as taking ownership of their journey into motherhood.

In 1956, Prunella Briance founded the Natural Childbirth Trust, later renamed the National Childbirth Trust (NCT) in 1961 (nct.org. uk). This charitable organisation aimed to address these shortcomings by providing practical and emotional support for expectant mothers through a network of volunteers. Activities included antenatal classes, breastfeeding workshops, postnatal sessions, jumble sales and other social events. Women were encouraged to believe they were not just passive recipients of care, but active participants in a two-way process, thus establishing a balance of power between mother and midwife. Yet again, maternity care was ahead of its time, with other medical specialities introducing patient support groups decades later. However, mounting pressure due to midwifery staff shortages, which led to disruption in community-based service, meant that in many cases the only real continuity offered to pregnant women was via the NCT. Over the decades, valid campaigns such as challenging to use of stirrups, shaving pubic hair and enemas were replaced by more assertive messages around empowerment to keep the organisation fresh and relevant. Increased demand for pregnancy-related information allowed many similar organisations to be established, but the NCT remains the largest provider with more than 100,000 parents attending classes each year.

However, the contribution made by the NCT pales into insignificance when compared with the internet, which, in the past 20 years, has brought about an explosion of websites, blogs, chatrooms, Facebook groups and so on. Endless streams of information from these sources have rendered older female family members and experienced frontline midwives virtually obsolete in the pregnancy and childbirth narrative. Their advice is easily overlooked in favour of 'evidence' from online sources accessible 24/7. These often encourage unvetted opinion and continuous live interaction, prompting today's clients to ruminate obsessively about every detail of their pregnancy and birth. Many spend much of the day, and night, surfing the internet almost as if it were a full-time job. In the past, women had to work hard to obtain information; now they are being bombarded by huge volumes of it, with links and hyperlinks that take them down rabbit holes on issues they never knew existed. No opportunity for advertising and marketing pregnancy-related products is wasted, putting financial pressure on young families keen to procure the latest 'must-have' items. Those not keeping up with the latest trends feel inadequate and left out, as if society has judged them to be unfit parents.

So powerful is the online communication space that, within weeks, a 'new' concept that previous generations of mothers seemed to get by without considering can achieve great prominence. Examples include placental location and colostrum harvesting. The internet has become the primary source of truth and, because this platform thrives on dramatic stories, extremely rare or quite simply fabricated events 'go viral' quickly and easily. YouTube videos of malformed babies, babies getting stuck in labour, gruesome images of caesarean deliveries, accounts of women nearly bleeding to death, babies being kidnapped from postnatal wards or mothers jumping off ten-storey buildings due to postnatal psychosis all make for great stories. Impressionable clients begin to think these events are the norm, but even for more pragmatic or sceptical types, it is unlikely that bombardment with such 'information' and imagery will make for a calm, confident approach to dealing with the challenges that lie ahead.

Despite this limitless amount of information, the painful reality for both clients and frontline staff is that, in the event or an unfavourable outcome, there are cries of 'The midwife didn't warn me this could happen' or 'How was I to know, I am not the professional?' or 'Why did the doctor not discuss these options?' When disaster strikes, none of these sources of information matter, none are accountable for their messages, none can provide practical help. How is it that today's clients are so well 'informed' on the one hand and yet seem to understand so little on the other? The answer is simple. It is because the deluge of pregnancy-related information available today fails to alert clients to the real issues. The challenge in navigating modern maternity care is no longer obtaining information; it is difficult not to be engulfed by it. Instead, the real skill is the ability to distil, preserve and digest the very, very tiny amount that is accurate and relevant and, crucially, to place it in context. This requires attention to detail, a healthy suspicion of the 'facts', the ability to be inquisitive and think critically, and a liberal exploration of alternative explanations for any given phenomenon. In other words, getting correct and meaningful pregnancy-related information today has become the domain of the emotionally composed and intellectually advantaged, leaving the rest behind as ill-fated believers.

Maternity care misinformation and disinformation pose problems on several levels. First, no one likes to consider themselves gullible, so continuing to act in accordance with preconceived ideas or seeking out further information to reinforce one's firmly held beliefs becomes commonplace. Second, today's midwives and obstetricians cannot politely but firmly disabuse mothers-to-be of any preconceived notions because they will be accused of 'not listening' or 'not placing mother and baby front and centre of care provision', so any communication that might be perceived as dismissive or contradictory is avoided in favour of rolling with the 'patients know best' philosophy of modern care. Third, frontline staff do not have sufficient clinic time to engage in meaningful discussions, so self-censorship minimises clinic overruns and complaints. Unfortunately, my view is that failure to challenge some of the information provided to maternity clients has undeniably contributed to poor outcomes.

It is tempting to think that in among the tsunami of information, at least a droplet or two of sensible advice might trickle through, but even the most robustly validated information is of no value without context, otherwise it can appear falsely reassuring or unnecessarily concerning. For example, take the RCOG-approved patient information on VBAC (RCOG 2016), which quotes an overall success rate of more than 75 per cent. This sounds optimistic, but because the range of possible outcomes is vast and without individualised counselling based on past obstetric history, the overall information is of no value. Non-contextualised information is interpreted subjectively and may influence decision making in an illogical way. For example, the nationally quoted risk of 6 per cent of sustaining a third-degree tear for first-time mothers (RCOG 2015) can cause one client carrying a smallish baby with a well-engaged and optimally positioned fetal head low in the pelvis to be anxious enough to request delivery by elective caesarean section, whereas another who is ten days overdue with a large baby in the occipito-posterior position negotiates with her midwife for a further four days before agreeing to induction of labour because she thinks her risk of having a third-degree tear is 'only' 6 per cent. Conflicting information also creates anxiety. For example, mothers often ask 'How long should I breastfeed for? Some sources say six months, others say three months is good enough' or 'I know I must lie on my left side but when I wake up and find myself on my back, have I harmed my baby?' or 'I know I must not eat soft cheese, but some sources say it is OK as long as it is heated – is that true?' or 'I was told ankle swelling is normal but then I read the internet I am told I should be checked for blood clots – what do I do?'

The day of delivery is often perceived by clients as the most important day of the whole pregnancy. Information accrued over the preceding months must be put into practice; events are often stage-managed like a live theatre performance. Props include pillows, birthing balls, aromatherapy oils, water bottles and face sprays. Actions are scripted and, in some cases, clients become irritated if the birth partner shows hesitation, forgets their lines or misses their cue. 'Make sure the MW does delayed cord clamping... 'Have you taken a video yet?' ... 'This is not the soundtrack he should be born to!'... 'What are the Apgar scores?'... 'Why is she not latching on?' Studies have shown that information that raises expectations and encourages overprepa-ration for this inherently unpredictable event has led to a steady rise in fretfulness and apprehension, especially among first-time mothers (Moujaes & Verrier 2021). Some midwives go as far as suggesting that non-stop bombardment with advice and anecdotes causes a constant low-grade anxiety that contributes to a rise in postdates pregnancies, less efficient labour, problems establishing breastfeeding and may even affect bonding, but there is no way of proving this.

Client choice

The main reason for providing information to clients is to enable them to exercise their right to choose. This is a highly charged topic (Glosswitch 2016), so I will discuss it purely from the perspective of personal observation.

As explained previously, after the establishment of the NHS in 1948, community midwives continued to provide the lion's share of maternity care, but by the late 1960s and early 1970s the service had become a hospital-based one. At that time, women were able to access contraception and legalised abortion, and new developments in pain relief for labour became increasingly popular, offering this generation far more choice. By the late 1970s and 1980s, many women were using epidural analgesia in labour, and with this the role of anaesthetists and obstetricians became more prominent. Around that time the 'active management of labour', a series of interventions designed to ensure that no first-time mother was in active labour for more than 12 hours, was gaining widespread traction. This practice was first introduced in Ireland in the 1960s by consultant obstetrician Kieran O'Driscoll (O'Driscoll et al 1973) but soon spread to the UK. Allowing mothers to drift on in labour for several days at a time was considered unkind, and shorter, more efficient labours became popular. The wide range of improved formula milk products also meant many mothers chose not to breastfeed. Motherhood was being redefined.

But the late 1980s and early 1990s brought about a backlash against the increasing medicalisation of childbirth. As discussed in Chapter 4, around this time the WHO recommended a maximum caesarean section rate target of 15 per cent across its 194 member countries, the UK average being around 20 per cent at that time. The anti-medicalisation effort in the UK was led by some pretty vocal consumer groups, aided by midwives who saw this wave of opinion as an opportunity to reclaim their rightful territory. This reignited midwifery dominance in this sphere of public discourse and resulted in the birthing narrative pivoting disproportionately towards 'natural' birth. Women were encouraged to actively choose this option, the same 'option' their mothers and grandmothers would have been presented with because in their time there was simply no alternative. Anaesthetic and obstetric interventions were framed as not only 'unnecessary' but in some cases 'unsafe'. Women were warned against the 'cascade of intervention' if they agreed to induction of labour or requested epidural analgesia. The message was clear: pregnancy and birthing were natural phenomena in which modern medicine played no part. But the problem with leaving things entirely to nature, as the wording might suggest, is that it would give us the same perinatal outcomes as those in the 1800s, when records first began, or indeed the same outcomes as occur in some of the most impoverished parts of the world today (see Chapter 2). It is unlikely that those who championed 'natural birth' so stridently in the late 20th century really wanted this. What they were probably aiming for was a commitment to achieve vaginal birth without an abundance of monitoring, drugs and operative assistance. Unfortunately, however, this legacy shaped behaviours in ways that continue to cause harm and distress decades later.

Let us look at the ultimate expression of client choice, the birth plan. In many ways committing birthing preferences in writing is both reasonable and rational. Clients recognise that on the day they may not be able to leisurely consider all that is on offer, and they may wish to avoid unnecessary repetition to different carers. What is striking though is that more than 90 per cent of these birth plans, supposedly a highly individualised account of preferences, say the same thing – partner present, keep the room quiet, low-level lighting, encourage free movement, client to remain upright so that gravity assists labour, do not offer epidural unless requested by the client, staff to discuss all options thoroughly with the client and birth partner, parents to be given time to consider all options, caesarean only if medically indicated, immediate skin-to-skin, delayed umbilical cord clamping, physiological delivery of the placenta, exclusive breastfeeding, baby not to be offered formula milk and so on. The 'natural birth' narrative has become so influential in the UK that most clients will wholeheartedly subscribe to it, such that their 'individualised' birth plan ends up looking just like everyone else's. Indeed, there are cut-and-paste options widely available on the internet where one simply enters one's partner's name in the empty field. In a liberal democracy, we are quick to mock countries in which institutions and organisations seek to control the thoughts and actions of their populations, yet slow to recognise similar behaviours operating in our own society. But how is it that the 'natural birth' message is so captivating? More fascinatingly, how come this message transcends most of life's usual barriers, such as social class, income bracket, educational attainment, religious beliefs or cultural values?

I do not pretend to know the answers to these questions, but it seems there is subconscious messaging at play that encourages some clients to equate this birthing ideal with being a 'good' mother and, of course, everyone wants to be that, whatever their background. I regularly care for clients who regard their ability to birth 'naturally' almost as a competition between their peers, wishing to prove they could progress further in labour compared with a friend or sister-in-law before asking for epidural analgesia, or endure a longer labour, or avoid instrumental delivery or caesarean section. Such interventions are for less good mothers, less dedicated, less self-sacrificing. Comments like 'well done' if a client managed to labour without using epidural analgesia or deliver a 9 lb baby unassisted after a 36-hour labour, and 'Never mind, better luck next time' if delivery was by caesarean, reinforce these beliefs. Parents sometimes shed tears of disappointment at caesarean deliveries, an event perceived as regrettable. This act of 'failure' is destined to be blamed for any subsequent problems with lactation, bonding, post-operative recovery or postnatal depression, and many go on to develop PTSD. And the contest continues after birth, with guilt and shame being an accepted part of postnatal life. Comments such as 'I don't have enough milk so I'm afraid I had to give her formula' are presented as an apology, an admission of defeat, rather than being framed for what it is – a caring mother who does not want her baby to go hungry. Pejorative lines of questioning from peers such as 'How come you gave up feeding your baby after just three months?' or disparaging comments such as 'Don't worry, it can take a while to lose that extra pregnancy weight' compound the sense of failure. The need to suffer, sacrifice oneself, feel guilty, compare yourself to others and tolerate judgement or criticism when you have fallen short of a preset ideal of motherhood are topics explored in depth in the compelling work of Eliane Glaser (Glaser 2021).

But these issues are not specific to motherhood; they are deeply ingrained in the female psyche. The same factors operate in the multi-billion-pound diet, makeup and fashion industries, all with a predominantly female clientele, all setting the bar at some imaginary and largely unachievable level, with an inherent understanding that falling below the mark means undeniable and inexcusable failure. The verdict is binary: you have either made it or you have not. And despite many businesses and services taking very welcome and long overdue steps to offer more inclusive examples or female representation in marketing and advertising, the criteria that need to be met to qualify as beautiful, fashionable or indeed a good mother remain disappointingly and damagingly narrow. I cannot imagine a world in which men would fall victim to such judgements to the same extent. Society is cruel to women and the consequences are often tragic – anxiety, depression, nervous breakdowns, anorexia and other eating disorders, and, specific to events around childbirth, birth trauma, postnatal depression and even suicide. It is estimated that 10–20 per cent of first-time mothers suffer from poor perinatal mental health (UK Government 2019) and postnatal PTSD is so common that most maternity units have set up birth trauma clinics (Birth Trauma 2024).

Of course, there are women who do not subscribe to the 'natural birth' narrative at all, and they often make very different choices and request intervention. Adverse media coverage and loss of faith in the maternity service are often cited as drivers for the increase in maternal requests for caesarean sections even when there are no medical indications, although the evidence for this is flimsy. One unforgettable birth plan simply stated 'I want staff to do whatever it takes to make sure my baby is healthy', which might sound unusually pragmatic, but this client had suffered an unexplained term stillbirth two years earlier. This was not a birth plan as much as it was an expression of hope, because when one has experienced such tragedy, notions of exercising choice or focusing on the birthing experience are unimportant in comparison.

For some clients, the intervention-free pregnancy and 'natural birth' narrative will align perfectly with their experience on the day, and one of the most telling findings of the 2022 CQC maternity care survey, which is almost never highlighted, is that those least likely to report shortcomings in maternity care were those who achieved unassisted vaginal birth. Achieving the 'gold standard' brings peace and contentment and negates the need to look for fault or apportion blame. For others, the intervention-free pregnancy and birth will be a far less good fit, but because the messages are so powerful many clients enter a state of denial and continue to force the fit even when all the evidence points to the contrary. For example, frontline staff will be all too familiar with the reactions of a client who cannot believe you are advising her that she is not suitable for a pool birth because her large uterine fibroids put her at increased risk of postpartum haemorrhage, or another whom you advised should consider induction of labour with continuous fetal heart rate monitoring as the baby has not grown for the past three weeks. On some occasions this has felt like telling a small child that Santa Claus does not exist. After they have recovered from the shock caused by this devastating news, then follows the negotiation – 'Can I have another scan?' or 'I will think about this and get back to you' or 'I would like to see another midwife/doctor'.

Requesting second opinions was almost unheard of 20 years ago, but it is part of everyday life today as public pressure mounts and frontline staff battle against continued accusations of closing ranks, dismissing patient concerns and failing to support alternative care pathways in accordance with client choices. Indeed, nowadays second opinions are often positively encouraged by frontline staff who feel they must share the responsibility of shattering a client's dreams with other carers. Despite calls for this to be embedded in routine NHS practice (Mills 2023), limited frontline staffing means that lack of easy access to multiple opinions may lead to further client frustration and, in an acute obstetric emergency, cause delays with potentially devastating consequences (Church 2023).

Increasingly, maternity clients 'shop around' to get the opinion they like best. Sometimes clients propose alternate care arrangements in semi-recognition of the problem – 'Can I have daily monitoring instead of induction of labour?' or 'Can I postpone the induction until next week because we are moving house?' Less experienced frontline staff are more likely to acquiesce to these demands and, in so doing, give the impression that induction of labour was not really that necessary in the first place. Similarly, 'Can I wait for another week before I start my medication?' may in truth simply serve to advance the disease process but may make the client feel better as they have gained the upper hand and frontline staff have been forced to compromise. Frontline staff know that pre-eclampsia left untreated today may become eclampsia tomorrow, but to forecast bad outcomes if advice is not followed is seen as threatening and denying clients the right to choose. Anecdotes aimed at undermining the views of professionals are common: 'Well, they told my sister she had a small baby, he was over 6 lb at birth and now my nephew is the tallest boy in the class.' Or every frontliner's favourite: 'They said I needed a caesarean because the baby was distressed but she came out in perfect condition, so I don't think I needed it after all.'

In essence, overemphasis on avoiding intervention with a view to achieving 'natural' birth has left clients ill prepared to cope with or agree to deviations from the seemingly one and only plan they are ideologically committed to. In recognition that most 'birth plans' do not go according to plan, there has been a conscious attempt to talk about 'birth preferences' instead, but there is little evidence that this change in wording softens the blow for mothers when events do not unfold as they imagined.

With some notable exceptions, almost all adverse outcomes in maternity care are the result of poor choices. Frontline maternity staff understand this all too well because their poor choices or bad decisions, erroneous actions or omissions are easily revealed by self-reflection, discussion with colleagues or incident investigations. They must be prepared to be challenged, justify their decisions and actions, be transparent about the part they played in the outcome, apologise to the patient and engage with corrective measures. But what if the client makes bad choices? What if the recommended course of treatment is declined only to find, in retrospect, that one should have complied with advice? What if harm occurs as a result of following advice obtained from a source propagating unsubstantiated or wrong information? It would seem only fair that the client, or other parties instrumental in her decision making, carry some responsibility. But this never happens. When cases go to external review, the witness statements of frontline staff often read as polar opposites to accounts by service users. For example, the frontline staff will have documented 'mother requested pushing for a further ten minutes as feels delivery is imminent', whereas the client's statement will read 'I had been asking for a caesarean section for several hours', corroborated of course by the birthing partner whose report always echoes, or even amplifies, hers.

Some client choices cause great unease among frontline staff such as the insistence on being seen only by the consultant in antenatal clinic, a choice often articulated forcefully or by those least in need of senior input. Occasionally, mothers decline male attendants, which is not only prejudicial but almost certainly a factor contributing to the gender imbalance in our speciality as male doctors have turned their backs on this discriminatory work environment. Sometimes the requests are nothing short of offensive and would not be tolerated in any other workplace, such as a client who refused to be attended to by a midwife wearing a hijab, or another who refused to be seen by a Black obstetrician, later writing in a letter of complaint that she 'had to wait for over two hours only to find that there was no one suitable' to attend to her. Disappointingly, this was followed by a letter of apology from the complaints manager and a prompt rescheduling of her appointment to coincide with the presence of an obstetrician whose appearance was more to her liking. Frontline staff cannot pick and choose whom they attend to and, quite rightly, they have a moral and professional obligation to care for everyone. Refusing to do so puts their professional registration at risk. Sadly, it seems that for a small group of maternity service users, any number of prejudices can thrive under the guise of 'patient choice'. That said, patient choice is often just an illusion, biased propaganda from a service wishing to model itself on the corporate sector. For example, only very limited choice can be exercised when booking appointments or procedures, and there is no real choice when it comes to which medicines are prescribed, whether there are cancellations or delays, which hospitals will accept in-utero transfers and so on.

Understanding risk and prioritising safety

If you ask most mothers what their main priority is, they will say they want a healthy baby, often followed by the curious statement 'It doesn't matter about me, as long as my baby is OK'. Clearly, both are important, and maternity is the only medical speciality where frontline staff look after at least two patients at any one time. They never have the luxury of concentrating on just one patient. This is an extraordinary privilege but what follows is that risk and safety concerns are multiplied accordingly, a fact that seems so obvious when presented in this way but is rarely taken into consideration when assessing the merits or needs of a functional maternity service. If stripped down to the bare bones, the mission is simple – to do whatever it takes to keep mothers and babies safe at all times. Any derogation from this basic principle, by any interested party, will cause problems.

Now, I totally accept that discussions with clients about risk and clinical safety are extremely dull. Concepts around 'risk' pose particular problems because this is not simply a matter of facts and figures. Far from it. If this were the case, clients would not make choices that seem mathematically illogical. For example, a client might avoid eating unpasteurised food despite the low probability of listeriosis then choose to attempt VBAC where the risk of harm is significantly higher. Another might choose to have an amniocentesis for extra reassurance despite a low probability trisomy 21 (Down syndrome) screening result yet opt for IA during labour. Risk perception among clients varies greatly according to a large number of factors, including educational attainment, social capital, past experience, personality, anecdote, strongly held religious or cultural beliefs and expectation, all of which influence clinical outcome. Many reports have highlighted disproportionately poor maternity outcomes in certain ethnic groups. Tragically, while the overall maternal mortality for the UK is 12.67/100,000, it is 12.2/100,000 for white mothers, 16.7/100,000 for Asian mothers and 28.2/100,000 for Black mothers (MBRRACE 2025). Similarly, while the overall stillbirth rate for England and Wales is 3.9/1000, it is 3.2/1,000 for babies born to white British mothers, 4.3-5.3/1,000 for babies born to Asian mothers, and 4.6-9/1,000 for babies born to Black mothers (ONS 2025). Independent national inquiries suggest this unacceptable situation is the consequence of unconscious bias and racism within maternity services, but undoubtedly there are multiple confounding variables at play such as the contribution of socioeconomic factors. Data reveals that maternal mortality is 10.25/100,000 in the most affluent 20 per cent of the population whereas it is 18.77/100,000 in the 20 per cent who are least affluent (MBRRACE 2025) and while there may be some overlap, it would be misleading to conclude that better maternity care for non-white British mothers alone is all that is needed to address the issues (Vousden et al 2024).

Let us start with the easy bit – the facts. In 1970, the caesarean section rate in England was 4 per cent, but it has steadily increased to 16 per cent in 1995, 20 per cent in 1999, 29 per cent in 2020, 39 per cent in 2022/3, and the latest data reports 42 per cent in 2023/2024 with only 46 per cent of mothers having spontaneous vaginal births (NHS Digital 2024) so it does not take much to realise that in today's NHS maternity service the intervention-free birth is experienced by a minority.

There are many reasons for these changes. Some are obvious, such as clients getting older, mostly through choice, as women prioritise careers before starting a family. Many older women require assisted conception and, although sex education at school concentrates on contraception and pregnancy avoidance, there is little mention of risks if pregnancy is deferred. For these women, pregnancies are medicalised from the start. The increased prevalence of chronic illnesses, such as type 2 diabetes, epilepsy, inflammatory bowel disease or other autoimmune diseases, can impact pregnancy. Some women have had medical procedures earlier in their lives that were not available to previous generations, such as cardiac surgery for congenital heart disease or kidney transplants, which mean they have survived into their reproductive years. Crucially, women in the UK today are far less fit, with 49 per cent entering pregnancy overweight or obese (Public Health England 2019). High body mass index (BMI) is associated with nutritional imbalance, vitamin D deficiency and increased risk of almost all pregnancy-related complications, including miscarriage, extremes of fetal growth, gestational diabetes, hypertension, pre-eclampsia, shoulder dystocia, stillbirth and venous thrombo-embolism (RCOG 2018). It is known that screening tests are less reliable in high BMI mothers and that surgical complications are more likely (Zozzaro-Smith 2014). Caring for obese clients poses practical challenges, such as ensuring availability of the appropriate equipment (for example, large blood pressure cuffs or operating tables designed for heavier weights), and moving and handling of these clients can be difficult, especially in an emergency. Other clients make choices that compromise outcomes such as smoking or use of illicit drugs.

But there are less obvious factors that feed into medicalised birth (Spendlove 2017). Frontline staff are less experienced and provide care that is far less intuitive and much more process driven. Staff shortages and fragmented working patterns make continuity of care impossible, which compounds concerns over error and blame. And while service users want autonomy and choice, they are also intolerant of uncertainty or failure.

Now for the complicated bit. Unfortunately for all three parties – service users, service providers and service organisers – the facts discussed above do not sit comfortably alongside the 'natural birth' narrative, which has resulted in what I call the 'expectation–reality mismatch'. The messages of yesteryear have not changed to reflect the demographic of today. This is dangerous for many reasons.

First, the wording 'natural birth' can cause upset because it makes clients who are unable to achieve it feel that operative vaginal delivery or caesarean section is somehow 'unnatural'. The even more toxic phrase 'normal birth' is often used interchangeably with 'natural birth' to describe spontaneous vaginal birth but subliminally suggests that all alternatives are somehow 'abnormal'. This means that over 50 per cent of all women in the UK today have 'abnormal' births. Really?

Second, it results in a tendency for information to be withheld, presented subjectively or sugar coated to avoid upset. For example, clients often report that antenatal course facilitators do not talk about epidural analgesia, or give it just a cursory mention, because focusing on this 'only encourages mothers to ask for it'. How can something that more than 60 per cent of clients use during their birth not be discussed? In one memorable case, a mother reported being left in tears because the whole class ganged up on her when she declared that she was not planning to breastfeed her baby. 'Why on Earth would you poison your baby with formula milk?' they cried. She was HIV positive with a high viral load, so had been advised not to breastfeed, but she did not wish to share this with her class. Her understanding and acceptance of risk made her feel like an outsider. Difficult issues that deserve careful consideration such as VBAC are substituted by patient information leaflets or directing clients towards various internet sites that provide bland, non-committal and depersonalised information. Messages can be misleading because they encourage clients to believe they can have their cake and eat it. For example, the so-called 'mobile epidural', which allegedly provides all the pain relief yet allows delivery on all fours or standing up: when faced with the reality of IV access, BP monitoring, feeling faint, weak legs and a urinary catheter, the mother soon realises she has been conned. Same for the so-called 'gentle caesarean section' where the baby supposedly 'crawls up' the mother's chest to 'seek out the milk', another empty promise that often backfires. It is wrong to offer false hope because in so doing one precludes intelligent, balanced discussions from taking place. This is why so many women who end up having inductions of labour, epidural analgesia or being delivered by unplanned caesarean section often know very little about these procedures other than that they are unwanted.

Third, pursuit of the 'natural birth' ideal can cause frontline staff to alter their behaviour in a way that may unintentionally cause harm. This is especially true for midwives, who are more likely to feel conflicted or disloyal if they do not support maternal choice. For example, when interpreting a CTG recording a midwife may subconsciously raise the threshold at which she calls for medical review. There is a tendency to seek reassurance, downplay risk or dismiss borderline findings as variants of normal, but these compassionate acts are often the root cause of many poor outcomes. Obstetric pathology is rarely acute or unpredictable. This statement might surprise those who have read serious incident reports or cases in independent national inquiries because these focus on failure to recognise an acute problem, escalate to seniors or take timely action in a crisis. However, most (definitely not all) so-called 'acute' conditions have a prodrome which is visible hours, weeks, often months before disaster strikes. It is often easier not to raise issues proactively because telling a client there might be problems ahead can be stressful for both parties, especially if all ends well, as it so often does. Remember, even if mothers receive no care, mostly all will be fine.

I believe that fear of being accused of causing unnecessary alarm or doom-mongering has resulted in a culture of caregiving in which safety is taken for granted and proactive care aimed at averting disaster is forfeited in favour of reactive emergency care. Retrospective analyses of cases of intrapartum birth asphyxia almost always conclude that there were several time points earlier in the labour at which a more proactive approach could have resulted in a better outcome and, while it was the terminal fetal bradycardia that prompted delivery by emergency caesarean section in the end, it was the meconium liquor, the slow progress due to occipito-posterior presentation, the pyrexia in labour and the prolonged use of oxytocin in the 36 hours prior to delivery that had all been 'normalised' to avoid conflict with the client's preferences. Despite my many years in clinical practice, it is still surprising to me how many clients, poorly informed of the real medical risks and ideologically committed to pursuing 'natural birth' despite unfavourable circumstances, are taken aback when the obstetric team come in following the sounding of the emergency buzzer and scramble to get her to the operating theatre as soon as possible, how frightened she looks when the specialist registrar tries hurriedly to obtain written consent for caesarean delivery, how little she will remember of the facts and figures quoted to her, and how awful she and her partner will feel as they watch the neonatal crash team deliver chest compressions to their apparently lifeless newborn. They are aware of the nightmare unfolding before them, but not yet aware that this is just the beginning of their troubles.

In the next few weeks and months, they will reflect upon their care, read around the issues, discuss their case with support groups, perhaps even seek medicolegal advice. Now, albeit too late in the day, they have meaningful information to hand, now they understand the risks, now they see what choices they should have made. All those messages from external sources about avoiding induction because it was 'unnatural', choosing instead to await spontaneous labour, the reassurances that going overdue was 'normal' for first-time mothers, practising those breathing exercises, the request for soft lighting, which meant that the meconium was not clearly seen, the disappointment felt when they were denied delayed cord clamping as the baby emerged floppy and unable to breathe, the inability to do skin-to-skin because the baby required full resuscitation and intubation. It all comes back to haunt them time and time again. The staple diet of advice aimed at achieving that perfect 'natural' birth they were fed throughout pregnancy now makes them feel sick; they are incandescent with rage. They have endless questions swirling around in their heads and all the answers are unsatisfactory.

Last, and perhaps most damagingly for the future of maternity care, widespread consumption of the singular 'natural birth' narrative has meant the service continues to be shaped according to service users' wishes rather than their *needs*. This is why, over the years, funding has been ploughed into birth centres while most UK maternity units struggle with limited obstetric theatre capacity, resulting in cancellation of elective caesareans and delays when multiple cases need urgent operative intervention simultaneously. With a transfer rate to obstetric units of 45 per cent for mothers who choose to birth at home and 36–40 per cent for those who choose to birth in a midwifery unit (Hollowell et al 2015) and the national caesarean section rate continuing to rise, it is difficult not to conclude that these service development choices represent serious errors of judgement. Thus, the mission of doing whatever it takes to keep mothers and babies safe at all times becomes ever harder to accomplish.

Conclusion

Good quality maternity care is dependent upon a partnership between those responsible for delivering it (service providers and service organisers) and those who need to access it (service users). It is my view that a functional maternity service requires service users to play their part by:

+ recognising that most mass-produced pregnancy-related information is of poor quality at best and misleading at worst
+ being willing to reject birthing narratives that sound too good to be true
+ understanding that standardised information may not be applicable in every case and that pregnancy is an individual journey
+ appreciating the enormous pressures frontline staff are working under and that 'the Service' is largely shaped by people in back-office roles
+ questioning critically whether there might be ulterior motives, which means that some client choices are well supported, for example the historical drive to bring down the caesarean section rate, while others are not
+ appreciating that pregnancy, and especially labour, are dynamic processes in which things can often change very quickly so it is best to be prepared for all eventualities
+ remembering that in maternity, as in all walks of life, choices have consequences
+ focusing on the end game – healthy mothers and healthy babies.

One of the most disturbing issues raised in independent national inquiries is how much resistance service users face when they wish to raise concerns. In the next chapter, I will discuss this in relation to all three parties.

When things go wrong: representation and the battle for improvement

Introduction

Many independent national inquiries undertaken over the past two decades were eventually, almost reluctantly, commissioned after grieving parents had fought for years to obtain answers to their own tragic cases (UK Parliament 2013; Woods 2022). In the meantime, avoidable disasters continued to occur. In a taxpayer-funded organisation that is supposedly striving to improve standards all the time, one would assume that all interested parties should have the benefit of accurate, fair and balanced representation so that each side can put forward their concerns and then work collectively towards the common aim of improved clinical outcomes long before an independent national inquiry is instigated. In this chapter, I will discuss how and by whom each of the three main stakeholders are represented when things go wrong, how easy it is for them to raise issues and how their grievances are dealt with.

The maternity service user

There are, in theory, a number of potential routes for a service user to raise concerns.

Become a patient representative

Patient representatives affiliated to NHS organisations are usually articulate and opinionated but, in my opinion, they rarely represent the wider group demographically and often vanish from the scene once their particular concern has been addressed. Their methods commonly range from relating overly personal anecdotes at meetings to pointed criticisms of certain frontline staff and, in recent years, stirring opinion on social media, which is now the preferred platform for anyone wishing to provide feedback. While these roles are well supported by service organisers (NHS England 2023), there are rarely tangible long-term improvements because remedial action requires more than temporary, sympathetic head nodding. In contrast, grief-stricken parents who set up external charities and action groups are likely to raise awareness more widely, although whether this translates into better future outcomes remains unclear.

Make a formal complaint

The NHS complaints policy is well established (NHS England 2024) and offers several points of contact. These include the Patient Advisory Liaison Service (PALS), which is usually situated at the entrance of most hospitals but rarely staffed so most complaints are submitted online. Patients can also contact their Healthwatch representative or direct their complaint to the latest version of the commissioning group or local authority. There is also the NHS Complaints Advocacy Service, or the Parliamentary and Health Service Ombudsman or Local Government and Social Care Ombudsman, if the complaint centres around community care.

The sheer volume of complaints means that most trusts employ complaints managers to respond. In most cases, the patient will receive a bland cut-and-paste letter expressing how sorry the trust is that they experienced such difficulties and that their case will be thoroughly investigated. Updates are slow and usually require chasing. Eventually, an email is sent containing stock phrases albeit with carefully inserted names to feign personalisation. It starts by thanking the client and relatives for their patience then outlines the results of the investigation. A list of lessons learnt is provided and reassurance given that procedures have been put in place to prevent recurrence.

The letter concludes with thanking the client and relatives for raising the issues and offering the opportunity for further discussion should there be ongoing concerns. These communications might appease some but leave others feeling 'processed' (Talwar & Doherty 2025).

Litigation

It is an absolute given that when a mother or baby suffers avoidable harm as a result of negligent care provided by NHS staff, they must have the right to instruct solicitors, who should in turn have easy access to the records to enable the case can be scrutinised. If breach of duty *and* causation are confirmed, the client and family should be offered compensation. Over the decades, the number of medical malpractice claims against the NHS has risen steadily, and although obstetric claims make up 'only' 13 per cent of the total, the value of those claims is around 57 per cent of the total payments (NHSR 2024). Accessing litigation lawyers is easy and efficient with 'no win, no fee' law firms advertising openly in many healthcare settings. In 2013, qualified one-way cost shifting was introduced for personal injury claims, guaranteeing that in all but the most exceptional cases, 'losing' claimants would not bear the defendant's costs, so clients and relatives are able to file cases knowing that the ball is firmly in their court. In practice, this has meant that even hopeless cases can run to advanced stages in the litigation process, racking up the trust's defence bill, which is ultimately taxpayers' money.

But with so little at stake, any service user who has the patience and stamina to endure the protracted legal proceedings will do well out of this system because, apart from the obvious enticement of a potential financial settlement, there is one other very worthwhile reward, namely a genuine, individualised and objective analysis of the care provided. When expert witnesses write their reports, they have no personal knowledge of, or vested interest in, the case. They do not work with the people who provided care, they have no connection to the trust in which care was provided, they have not met the mother or her family. Their analysis is free from the constraints of the trust-imposed tick-box maternity risk management exercise and falls outside the restricted terms of reference of HSIB/MNSI investigations. They are granted the freedom to express their genuine and unadulterated opinion because they are writing for the civil court, and their report cannot be altered to comply with the interests of healthcare commissioners or healthcare regulators. Unsurprisingly, these reports often reveal considerable shortcomings in previous in-house investigations or so-called 'independent' investigations by HSIB/MNSI. At long last, the service users get what they wanted all along: a sincere, honest and open account of the quality of care. Finally, everyone knows what perfect care would have looked like.

It is fair to say that no parent would prefer a financial settlement over a damage-free delivery, and although the money may soften the blow, it does not mean that justice is always dispensed. Some clients bring about poorly substantiated or even vexatious claims by writing fantastical and entirely subjective accounts of the horrors of their care, often vilifying one person while lavishing praise on another to give the impression of fairness and balance. At the opposite end of the spectrum, there are cases where care has been nothing short of appalling and service users have been subjected to the worst dereliction of duty by frontline staff, but because the case ended in stillbirth or neonatal death rather than long-term disability, claimant lawyers do not consider them of sufficient financial value to litigate over. Grim as it may be, partial redress in these cases is often achieved by a coroner's investigation but that provides scant consolation and little, if any, compensation for distressed parents and the wider family.

The maternity service provider

Broadly speaking, frontline workers can raise concerns or request representation internally from their employing trust or via external professional bodies.

Internal representation

Line manager

The first port of call for a frontline worker who has workplace concerns is, in theory, their line manager. Their physical absence and unwillingness to answer emails will be the first hurdle to overcome. Action is only likely if insignificant sums of money and minimal effort are required. In my experience, problems related to patient safety or poor clinical outcomes often receive polite nods and the promise of 'looking into the matter', often code for kicking problems into the long grass.

Senior management

A brave frontliner may choose to bypass their immediate line manager and go to someone more senior in the organisation. This can be a risky strategy. It has long been recognised that the plight of whistleblowers within the NHS maternity services is a very sad one (Thomas 2021; Allen 2020; Lintern 2021a). When Dr Catherine Hillman, a consultant obstetrician at Worcestershire Royal Hospital, posted her concerns about patient safety on social media, she was asked by her managers to withdraw her remarks. She refused, only to find her message had not only been withdrawn but replaced with another message supporting the changes introduced that had caused compromises in patient care in the first place, prompting Dr Hillman to resign. Ultimately, these events resulted in the downgrading of the maternity unit's rating, despite the managers' efforts to avoid this, even at the cost of losing a senior member of staff (Lintern 2021b).

It may seem odd to those outside the service that, despite the widespread appointment of so-called 'freedom to speak up guardians', a key recommendation of the Francis Inquiry into the mistakes at the Mid Staffordshire NHS Foundation Trust in 2013 (Francis 2013), the treatment of whistleblowers in the NHS still presents insurmountable problems. This is because these so-called 'guardians' are the very same people who sit on interview panels, conduct annual appraisals, are instrumental in clinical risk management processes, undertake exit interviews and write staff references. In short, they are in the perfect position to ensure not too much fuss is made about anything that might cause 'inconvenience'. Their version of the truth always wins because the fox is left in charge of the chicken coop. The individual wishing to raise issues usually backs down and is left with those three familiar options – put up with their lot, move to another maternity unit where things are unlikely to be better given the endemic nature of the rot, or leave the profession altogether. Independent inquiries into maternity care often describe a culture of acceptance among NHS staff working in underperforming units or paint a picture of indifference and resignation, but, in my view, it is far more complicated and insidious than that.

External organisations

Some staff feel morally obliged to raise issues despite the hurdles they face or the price they are forced to pay. Having had no joy through internal channels, they may try external organisations.

Royal colleges and professional unions

A midwife might attempt to contact the RCM which, apart from its primary role in education and training, also provides legal advice, representation and assistance in matters of employment. Alternatively, they might engage a nursing union such as UNISON, should they be a member, but their focus is often restricted to matters relating to conditions at work or remuneration. For obstetricians, the RCOG will not help as it exists purely to promote learning, research and continuing professional development. There is no shortage of training materials, courses and clinical guidelines emanating from this organisation, which prides itself on taking a neutral position in virtually all tricky matters. RCOG communications are efficient, predictable, polite and above all, non-committal. For example, the RCOG is quick to 'welcome the findings' of independent national inquiries and always 'looks forward to working in partnership with other organisations to address the issues', giving the impression that all staff need to do is educate and train themselves out of a little spot of bother. To many this seems an absurdly light approach to a toxic national storm, but the RCOG prioritises fundraising to maintain the organisation's reputation as a world leader on the international stage of women's healthcare, hoping that no one will ask too many questions about what is happening in maternity units back in the UK.

Then there is the British Medical Association (BMA, bma.org.uk) for obstetricians who are members. This organisation was established in Victorian times and purports to represent doctors and medical students largely in matters of employment, contractual obligations and remuneration, and it is the closest thing doctors have to a trade union. In postwar Britain, when the introduction of the NHS was being hotly debated in Parliament, the BMA proved to be a major irritant to the incumbent governments of the day because their members objected to being subsumed by the civil service, arguing that they were answerable only to the needs of their patients and not those of the then Ministry of Health. Members feared that the bureaucracy associated with being an employee of the state would choke off their professional autonomy (The National Archives 1948): a fear that was very real and, as history has proven, quite legitimate. Ultimately, the BMA was defeated not because the concerns of its members were without justification, but because it failed to propose a viable alternative for a more accessible healthcare service at a time when the prevailing winds of change were blowing strongly across a nation hoping to rebuild itself after the ravages of World War Two.

Traditionally, the BMA has cried off or sat on the fence over difficult issues and has often been seen as an archaic and stuffy organisation. In recent years, it has attempted greater involvement in key issues such as the negotiations around setting up of the seven-day service in 2015, but failure to address junior doctors' concerns ultimately led to strike action in 2016; doubtless the thin end of the wedge for further strikes in subsequent years. After the Covid pandemic, the BMA reported on the negative impact this had on frontline staff (BMA 2024a), but few doctors I have spoken to recall the organisation lobbying the DHSC for vital supplies to protect workers at the time. During the strikes of 2023 and beyond, which were ongoing at the time of writing, its leaders became uncharacteristically vocal about pay restoration for resident doctors in England (BMA 2024b), but it was the BMA which had allowed the below-inflation pay awards to continue unchallenged for the preceding 30 years. A particular gripe in maternity care, this being inherently a round-the-clock speciality, is the lack of provision for speciality-specific remuneration and this has led to poor support for the BMA among obstetricians.

Professional registering body

The most serious concerns about an individual's practice may result in a referral to their professional registering body, the Nursing and Midwifery Council for midwives and the General Medical Council for doctors.

The NMC has an important role in upholding public confidence in the nursing and midwifery profession, but it is a troubled organisation and was subject to a review in 2012, which found major weaknesses, including confusion over regulatory purpose, lack of strategic vision, poor working relationships, financial incompetence and a culture of damaging hierarchy (Council for Healthcare Regulatory Excellence 2012). The main grievances voiced by frontline midwives seem to centre around the organisation's penchant for predetermined judgement, and cases referred to the NMC are widely perceived as poorly assessed, inadequately scrutinised, never placed in context of general working practice. More than a decade later, reports of concealment of failures to act in cases of rogue nursing practices suggest things have not improved (Thomas 2024). If this sounds familiar, it may be because many of the individuals occupying key roles in this organisation are drawn from management backgrounds and have 'experience' in clinical risk, staff management or handling of complaints. The organisation they are affiliated to may have changed but their mentality and style of working have not.

Sadly, doctors fare no better. The GMC has historically controlled entry onto the register of practising doctors in the UK and had the power to suspend or remove members who are deemed unfit to practise. Following the unveiling of the horrendous series of killings over several decades by Dr Shipman in 2000, the GMC introduced a revalidation programme, and since then all doctors have been required to demonstrate their fitness to continue practising by taking part in annual appraisals, keeping an up-to-date e-portfolio, reflecting on cases where care could have been better and having an agreed annual personal development plan. If the information submitted to the responsible officer meets the required standards, the licence to continue practising is extended for a further five years, conditional upon continued annual appraisals.

The GMC runs regular workshops to remind doctors of their duties and code of conduct, but I am afraid to say that attendance at these leaves no one in any doubt that the view of this organisation is that every doctor is just another Dr Shipman waiting to be weeded out. Like all other professions, we have, and always will have, crooks, rogues and downright evil people in our midst, and these individuals understandably attract much media coverage and public outrage. But they form a tiny minority, and misrepresentation of the vast, well-meaning majority is spiteful and wounding to our profession. Frequent changes in the GMC's strapline are evidence of this organisation trying to project a less hostile approach to doctors: 'Protecting patients, guiding doctors' became 'Regulating doctors, ensuring good medical practice', then 'Working with doctors, working for patients', and lately 'Every

Voice Counts'. Whether appraisal and revalidation are useful screening tools for detecting the evil, incompetent or dangerous is debatable. Many doctors subsequently found guilty of truly awful crimes long after Shipman were regularly appraised and all seemed well. Some believe that appraisal does at least assist formative educational and professional development, although many experienced appraisers will be aware of anecdotal evidence that this process is used as a tool for blame, bullying or exclusion.

One might think that an organisation so proud of maintaining high moral standards would be beyond reproach, but the GMC has been criticised for the accusatory manner in which it conducts investigations which are thought to be instrumental in the extraordinarily high suicide rate among doctors undergoing investigation (GMC 2022; Rimmer 2023). In 2021, following an employment tribunal case against the GMC by a consultant urologist (Karim v GMC 2021) a UK court declared that, among its many other failings, the GMC was 'infected with racism' (Dyer 2021). Another example where the GMC did not do itself any favours was the case of Dr Hadiza Bawa-Garba, a specialist registrar in paediatrics, who was found guilty of manslaughter of a six-year-old boy under her care in 2015 (Bawa-Garba v GMC 2018). The circumstances surrounding the boy's death make for grim reading and it was widely acknowledged that his care was far from perfect, but the case sparked a public debate about the context in which medical mishaps occur. On the day of this tragic and, unquestionably, avoidable event, the unit was trying to manage multiple high-risk cases with a dire lack of frontline staff. It is impossible not to feel sorry for all parties, but it was the court's use of material Dr Bawa-Garba kept in her retrospective reflective notes to secure a conviction that most angered the medical profession. Dr Bawa-Garba's initial appeal was denied in 2016, and her name was removed from the medical register, but in 2018, a second appeal, widely supported by the medical profession, resulted in her name being restored to the register.

For many doctors, a particularly irksome annual event is receipt of the email notifying them of the exorbitant charges this organisation will levy in the forthcoming year for the privilege of compulsory membership in return for being treated with what they feel is utter disdain. In recent years, the GMC has bent over backwards to project a softer image as evidenced by pointedly inclusive language in recent Good Medical Practice Guides (GMC 2024), but from what I have seen support among many frontline staff remains lukewarm, and ongoing concerns about failures to represent the interests of the profession fairly have prompted the BMA to call for the creation of a new regulator (BMA 2025).

Legal representation

Allegations of clinical malpractice raised against frontline staff are a fact of everyday life now and, just like service users, service providers are entitled to legal representation. NHS trusts that are members of the CNST assume the role of named legal defendants so individuals contracted by them are indemnified. Additionally, midwives can get protection via RCM membership and obstetricians may choose to be a member of a medical defence organisation.

When notified of potential litigation, frontline staff are required to write a witness statement describing their involvement in the case using medical records to supplement their recollection of events. The introduction of electronic medical records, which was heralded as the panacea to all NHS problems, hardly ever provides better information than 'old-fashioned' paper notes because of data gaps, unsaved entries, underpopulated fields and the fact that most information is uploaded retrospectively. Many litigation cases are settled based on the quality of documentation being used as a proxy for substandard care. The deeply flawed clinical safety strategies discussed in Chapter 5 make for rich and easy pickings when litigation lawyers search for evidence of breach of duty and usually causation follows without too much difficulty. Following a landmark ruling in 2015 (Montgomery v Lanarkshire Health Board 2015), in most cases the UK law allows for clinical risk to be defined subjectively and retrospectively by the patient. This situation is compounded by the fact that most frontline staff have no appetite for conflict and maternity managers generally consider throwing the legal hounds a carcass or two a small price to pay for continuing to project a positive image of the service. Every NHS trust is cash strapped, so many do not have dedicated legal representatives and if they do, these individuals are in short-term positions often doing pro bono work until they gain some basic experience. Instructing experienced defence solicitors is costly and the imperative to save money results in quick settlements, often involving what many frontline staff consider disproportionately generous sums of money. Even if advice from the RCM or medical defence organisations is sought, frontline staff should be under no illusion that the emphasis will be on anything other than prompt settlement.

The maternity service organiser

Unlike the patient desperately seeking information or redress, or the frontline worker who is all too often left dissatisfied, perplexed or easily sacrificed, maternity service organisers are never formally impacted by an adverse event. Their roles are overarching and their strength in numbers grants them the ability to evade direct accountability for any shortcomings. Generally, they prefer not to raise concerns in case this suggests a disorganised or weak service. Unlike the other two parties, they are not represented as individuals, but rather as a collective. In the unlikely event that managers are asked to comment on an adverse incident, they will usually position themselves firmly behind the service user – and thus by default against frontline staff – and respond in the form of reassurances often delivered in the third person. For example, 'causes for concern have been identified and actions are in place to avoid recurrence'. By the time most cases come to judgement, they have almost certainly moved on several times over and thus distanced themselves from the problem.

Conclusion

From the examples I have given here, it's clear that raising concerns about the quality of NHS maternity care meaningfully and dealing with the problems effectively will only occur when:

+ concerns of service users *and* service providers are taken seriously
+ independent reviews of adverse incidents are truly independent
+ incentives to conceal problems are removed
+ all parties place good clinical outcomes at the top of their list of priorities.

Unfortunately, because none of these are properly in place, the net result is a maternity care system that is broken. I will discuss the consequences of this in the next chapter.

8

The consequences of a broken maternity service

Introduction

In the preceding chapters, I have sought to convey how changes in training, sheer workload, de-professionalisation and lack of managerial support have negatively impacted the ability of frontline staff to provide an effective service. I have also discussed how misinformation, disinformation, hyperbolic media coverage of adverse events, social pressures and anachronistic messages have left service users in a confused, conflicted and distrustful state. And I have given examples of how management-driven priorities have come to dominate all aspects of maternity service provision, most damagingly the adoption, implementation and misappropriation of clinical safety strategies that have failed to improve care. These factors have collectively and synergistically resulted in a broken maternity service, the key features and consequences of which are outlined below.

Mortality and morbidity

As discussed in Chapter 2, UK mortality data does not compare well with other developed countries but morbidity is also important. Permanent damage or disability in a mother or baby leaves a family having to relive the tragic events surrounding pregnancy and childbirth for years to come and manage the day-to-day reality of life-changing conditions. Contrary to the oversimplistic portrayal in the media, not all cases of mortality and morbidity are avoidable. But in a service that is inadequately staffed and poorly managed, and where formulaic investigations into adverse outcomes are fudged, deployed for alternative gain or written to placate service users, it has become almost impossible to distinguish avoidable versus unavoidable harm. Tragic outcomes are often an amalgam of the two, but enduring failures in analysing multiple confounding variables logically and systematically have resulted in the implementation of the wrong 'corrective' measures, so unsurprisingly, care does not improve.

Fear

Fear is experienced by all three groups. Service users experience fear or anxiety when they read about awful maternity outcomes. They lose faith if the service is slow, inefficient or staff seem uninterested, rushed, inattentive, inexperienced or indecisive. They desperately want guidance while still maintaining full autonomy, an impossible circle to square. Sources of information are plentiful, but none provide the individualised guidance they crave. Some choose to align themselves with health beliefs that are contrary to fact because the real facts are few and far between and presented poorly or threateningly. Others fall victim to mendacious propaganda. They are not aware that the apparent lack of guidance and direction from frontline staff is also a result of fear. If frontline staff had the confidence and time to demonstrate their knowledge and skills, they could engage with mothers more positively to secure their trust, the touchstone of safe care. Exchange of information could be factual, honest, free of nuances and management-driven steers and truly individualised so mothers can make better decisions.

In the current climate, frontline maternity staff are not free to practise autonomously because of a culture of fear and blame. Their professionalism has been curtailed, and many feel their primary objective is simply to survive the working day. Proposing vital or innovative changes to the service may look like criticism and stoke managerial objection, so best to stay silent. But to a mother, this sometimes comes across as staff who simply do not care – robots following processes, avoiding eye contact, ticking boxes on computer screens. Many frontline staff experience fear on a daily basis – fear of the reaction from parents if investigations reveal anomalous or unexpected findings (Johnson et al 2020), fear of being wrong, fear of appearing coercive or judgemental, fear of being accused of not providing patient-centred care, fear of acting outside the guidelines, fear of being named in a serious incident, fear of being investigated if something were to go wrong or if the patient expressed dissatisfaction, fear of being seen as unsupportive of the management. Many feel they are constantly treading on eggshells; some go as far as swapping shifts to avoid interacting with difficult colleagues. Others avoid decision making altogether and choose the 'clock in, clock out' style of working, but mistakes can also happen due to inertia, inactivity and disengagement.

Managers also experience fear. Fear that the service is not as good as they pretend it is, fear that cover-ups will be revealed or inadequate compliance data will result in a unit downgrade. Fear that promotion will be delayed or denied as a result.

The RCOG has reported that poor workplace behaviours are experienced by 23 per cent of midwives and 44 per cent of obstetricians (RCOG 2021), key contributors to disengagement, poor morale, sickness absence, employee turnover and lost productivity. One study estimated that fear costs the NHS a staggering £2.28 billion per annum (Kleine & Lewis 2019). Fear also results in 'organisational silence' (Pope 2018), which has dangerous repercussions because problems of the gravest kind can go unreported or passed over for years.

Waste of talent

The NHS is an organisation bursting with talent. Maternity care especially attracts dynamic, forward-thinking individuals willing to engage with a younger demographic, but recent pressures mean less and less of that talent is free to be unleashed for the good of patients.

Frontline staff are expected to routinely 'plug holes' in rosters and the service relies heavily on the good graces of its dedicated staff. A recent RCM report estimated that midwives give 100,000 hours of unpaid work to the NHS annually (RCM 2024). There is no obstetric-specific data, but NHS surveys show that 80 per cent of doctors regularly work unpaid overtime (Rimmer 2015). Based on attrition rates and the propensity of resident doctors to withdraw labour in recent years, it seems unlikely that the next generation will feel obliged to continue these sacrificial working practices, so this situation needs to be addressed now. The service must not continue to be dangerously over-reliant on bank, agency and locum staff because, while qualified to do the job on paper, their unfamiliarity with the surroundings and workings of the unit means they are overrepresented in poor maternity outcomes. It is deeply unfair to call upon these individuals in an hour of need and then blame them or declare them incompetent when disaster strikes. Every time these frontline staff are mentioned in incident investigations it is worth remembering they were only trying to keep a broken service functioning for a little while longer, but sustained improvements require stable midwifery and obstetric teams to genuinely take ownership of their part of the service.

The castigatory and vindictive approach to investigating poor outcomes also drives many talented individuals away. This 'one strike and you're out' system of analysing risk fails to take into account the complexities of multiple confounding factors or use of denominator data to lend context. For example, the practitioner with four post-operative complications in a year appears 'worse' than the one with only a single complication, but what if she has seven times as much work? Ironically, senior staff often have the highest complication rates because, understandably, they operate on the most complex cases. In one anecdotal case, the trust clinical risk lead stated, 'I have never seen a ureter tied off at caesarean.' A senior consultant ventured to suggest that anyone who had not unintentionally ligated a ureter at a caesarean had quite simply not done enough caesareans. Stunned silence filled the room. 'This is a perfectly well recognised complication of caesarean section, especially when undertaken at full cervical dilation as was the case here,' he went on to explain.

Inadvertent ureteric ligation is a correctable problem, usually with no long-term consequences, but in this case the mother got into trouble because she had the misfortune of needing delivery in the small hours of Friday morning and before her symptoms became apparent it was the weekend and no radiological imaging was available in that particular trust until the Monday morning, by which time she had developed septicaemia and required admission to the intensive care unit. She was not the victim of an incompetent surgeon so much as a service that, despite the aspirational soundbites, is far from functional 24/7, 365 days per week. It's perhaps not difficult to guess which of these 'lessons learnt' and 'corrective measures' were applied in this case: a) put pressure on the trust management to make 24-hour imaging for postoperative patients a priority; or b) send the two registrars involved, incidentally both very experienced, for extra surgical skills training. As if to rub salt into the wounds, the 'retraining' task was assessed as completed by the same clinical risk lead who, by her own admission, had 'never seen this problem'.

It is galling to have your professional reputation eviscerated by those with limited understanding of the situation but, in the current climate, when faced with speculation, rumour, gossip or doubt, the easiest course of action for any frontliner is to surrender to the process of being investigated, retrained or disciplined. The logical part of you might recognise that maternity risk management has been reduced to a rubber-stamping exercise, and it was just your turn to take one for the team. Close colleagues might rally around you and praise you for your ability to cope under pressure or work within such a chaotic system. You might try to convince yourself that you are entitled to occupy the moral high ground because at least you were there, attending to the patient in her hour of need, rather than sitting in an ivory tower casting judgement many weeks later. In this particular case, both registrars chose to leave: one pursued a career in medical education and the other went to work for a drug company. Two fewer for the frontline. What a waste. And with negative media coverage, anecdotal reports of ill treatment of staff and cynical accounts of working on the frontline, why should any talented young person want to train in midwifery or obstetrics today? Senior frontline staff have become conflicted because on the one hand, we loathe the feeling that we cannot inspire our gifted junior staff to stay on, strive for better and look forward to spearheading the service in years to come, but on the other we must admit their choices are based on sound judgements. They have looked down the barrel of the gun and stepped aside. Had our generation been faced with the same prospects all those years ago, we would surely have done the same.

Inefficient workflows

As I touched on in Chapter 4, workflows that don't work are a consequence of problems with staffing, poor IT systems and impractical layouts of maternity units.

Let me start from the client's perspective. After the mother has been registered for maternity care, future appointments are often pre-booked in an illogical order according to what is available on a clinic database. For example, it is not uncommon for a mother to attend an appointment to discuss mode of delivery, but the scan upon which the counselling is based is booked for three days later. Multiple appointments in one week are common – one day for a glucose tolerance test that screens for gestational diabetes, another day for a scan and a third day for a midwife appointment. This is not easy, especially for those who have jobs, carer's commitments or can barely afford the bus fare for a single round trip in a week, let alone three.

If a mother changes address during her pregnancy, direct referral from one maternity unit to another is not allowed due to maternity tariffing constraints forcing the mother to either self-refer online to her 'new' unit or request the GP to arrange transfer of care, which can take several weeks, resulting in disjointed care or omissions. Admission dates, times or locations are frequently noted down incorrectly, causing women to attend the wrong place at the wrong time, a particular problem for split-site units. Many patients find the automated 'did not attend' notification that follows irritating at best, or the sign of a dysfunctional service destined to keep letting them down at worst. Client confusion is further exacerbated by the interaction with countless members of frontline staff. Because most do not wear uniforms now, and when they do, they all look the same, service users are unsure who they are being cared for by or what their exact role or grade is despite the cheerful badges worn by most.

Clinic waiting times are variable but generally long, so women quickly learn to absolve themselves of any other commitment such as picking up their older children from school on the day of their appointment. Blood samples regularly get lost, especially if sent from the community clinics or GP surgeries. There are not enough staff to chase up results or have them communicated back to mothers with any degree of certainty, leaving many to access their own results via the trust maternity app and interpret them according to information from the internet. Lack of frontline staff also means that care is sometimes teasingly offered then withdrawn in what may seem like a cruel psychological game. For example, women who have their elective caesarean section cancelled (up to 20 per cent cases in some units due to a lack of frontline staff or theatre capacity) are often surprisingly understanding but find it hard to accept that they are advised to stay in hospital overnight so they 'don't lose [their] place in the queue'. They have done us a favour by accepting the limitations of our service, and in return they are detained unnecessarily at the taxpayers' expense. Similarly, women who are admitted for 'urgent' induction of labour due to concerns about blood pressure or inadequate fetal growth are perplexed by their two-day wait before the process commences, again mainly due to a lack of midwives.

Often NHS IT systems do not communicate with each other. For example, labour and delivery notes can be held on separate databases from imaging reports, which are on a separate database from the neonatal care records. Mothers' and babies' health records are often dissociated, and much of the information is incomplete because inadequate frontline staffing means that only mandatory fields are populated. Software systems lack inbuilt intelligence so, for example, it is entirely possible for a mother to be scheduled for a clinic appointment, an ultrasound scan and a caesarean section all at the same time on the same day. This duplication creates unfilled gaps in clinics, which is wasteful in an already stretched service. It can also, albeit unintentionally, cause considerable distress. For example, a mother who has suffered a stillbirth at 32 weeks continues to receive emails or text messages reminding her of appointments scheduled for later gestations because the software fails to recognise the pregnancy had concluded in the saddest of ways.

It is surprising how illogical the layout of some maternity units is. Co-location of clinical areas where close communication is important matters. For example, the obstetric ultrasound team needs to communicate regularly with obstetric day assessment staff, the maternity triage facility should be located next to the labour ward for efficient management of acute admissions, the postnatal ward should be near the neonatal unit to allow parents to visit their babies in the event of admission.

Inefficient workflows are not just an inconvenience for service users and frontline staff. They seriously impact the quality of care because service organisers cannot measure clinical activity or productivity, identify areas of increased risk, determine which areas are under-resourced and decide where increased investment will have the greatest impact.

Gaming the system

It is not difficult to game a broken system, and all three parties do this. Some service users engage with maternity care on their own terms. Missing appointments, turning up late and failing to comply with advice or medication cannot be challenged and are too easily forgiven and forgotten by frontline staff who prefer to work around problems rather than tackle them head on. Expert gamers use this to their advantage, for example by feigning abdominal pain to 'qualify' for an extra scan or flouting the rules around numbers of visitors or visiting times. During the Covid pandemic, some chose to 'shop around' for units that allowed attendance of birthing partners which, while socially understandable, made them appear oblivious to the risks of the virus or the resultant fragmented nature of their care.

A small group of mothers insist on 'out of guideline' care, where the mother presents frontline staff with an alternative care plan. This can include accepting some interventions but not others, rearranging the furnishings and equipment in a birthing room, altering the decor or allowing only some members of staff but not others to be involved in care provision. While frontline staff acknowledge that 'client choice' is an absolute right, they are also conscious of the impact this has on the care of other patients. Requests for 'out of guideline care' absorb huge resources as they require several consultations, recurrent explanations to which there is always a firmly held counternarrative and contingency plans which can compromise care for others. For example, cases where an operating theatre is 'reserved' for a specific case forcing others to be cancelled, or where special adaptations or concessions are made for a solitary case to meet exacting preferences.

Many frontline staff feel uncomfortable indulging a small minority at the expense of the majority, especially as these are often clients who will never be pleased no matter what is done to accommodate their wishes. This situation is made worse by the fact that alternative care pathways are usually sanctioned and supported by clinical managers who will never be present cometh the day of delivery, nor will they attend upon the mother in person, thus leaving frontline staff unfortunate enough to be on duty at the time to deal with these challenges unsupported. Patients with loud, demanding voices often achieve their aims within a service that is more concerned about proving it is providing patient-centred care than it is with fairness, equity and quality. Extreme entitlement and selfish, risky or offensive behaviours, while rare, are overlooked because frontline staff do not have the confidence, autonomy or managerial support to challenge them.

Frontline staff also game the system. I have discussed sickness and absenteeism already, but work avoidance is also a problem. This is when staff are physically present but make a minimal contribution. With so few maternity service managers leading by example and only too ready to turn a blind eye to underperforming or lazy staff, the 'somebody else's problem' approach to delivering care prevails, adding pressure to functional individuals who end up bearing the brunt. Clinical interventions or decisions are delayed until the next shift takes over, causing 'drifting' and mounting risk to mothers and babies. If maternity risk management was conducted in a meaningful way, it would show a disproportionate number of adverse outcomes occurring around handover times, a trend long recognised in obstetric litigation cases.

Because the frontline is an unhappy and unsupportive environment in which to work, tensions often run high and there are staff who frequently raise grievances against their colleagues. The sheer volume of these means that it is often impossible to distinguish real concerns about underperforming staff from opportunistic or frivolous allegations because they all need to be 'processed' in the same way. Even when the most serious safety concerns are raised, management processes often leave the person raising them feeling as if they are overreacting, or that they themselves are the perpetrator trying to pin blame on a colleague. The propensity for managers to allow incompetent and dangerous practices to continue operating under the radar is astonishing. Like many public service roles, most NHS contracts are long term, so short of summary dismissal in cases of gross misconduct, it is virtually impossible to terminate employment without substantial evidence of underperformance. Time-consuming investigations and meticulous documentation of all aspects of the case being brought against the individual are tedious undertakings. Then there is the need to offer retraining, performance management or even an alternative role. If all else fails, there are verbal and then written warnings. Managers do not have the appetite, organisational skills or longevity in post to follow these matters to their conclusion, so the gamer remains effectively untouchable.

In one busy maternity unit, a specialist midwifery practitioner took time off for sick leave due to pregnancy-related complications, followed by maternity leave for a year, briefly returned to work part time, then took bereavement leave following the death of her mother. After a short period back at work, she took time off for work-related stress, returning for a few weeks prior to resigning because she had been offered a job nearer to home. Carefully timed returns ensured she was on full pay for most of this time, but also meant that her job could not be advertised, so no replacement was appointed. Results were lost, patient care was compromised and well-meaning adminis-trative staff with no clinical background tried to help by attempting to prioritise and schedule clinical procedures. It was only after a client complained that another patient's blood test results had been filed in her records that the service was investigated and the full extent of how one individual had taken everyone for a ride was revealed. A service that relies on mistakes to address such poor behaviours is truly broken.

On a semi-positive note, there are other more 'honourable' examples of frontline staff gaming the system. For example, in 2004 the National Confidential Inquiry into Patient Outcome and Deaths (NCEPOD) classified surgical interventions according to clinical need (NCEPOD 2004) and decreed that category 4 procedures such as elective caesarean sections were not to be performed out of hours. Because many maternity units do not have a dedicated operating theatre and team for elective procedures, these are often squeezed in between emergency cases, but one of the 'tricks of the trade' is to prioritise in a way that reduces the risk of cancellation without increasing risk to patients. For example, the elective caesarean for breech is 'prioritised' at 2 pm, knowing that it will be easier to justify the out-of-hours undertaking of caesarean delivery in the mother with mild pre-eclampsia and a growth-restricted fetus but with a normal CTG at 36 weeks after 5 pm, although clearly a better solution would be to resource the frontline service properly in the first place.

Multiple examples of how maternity managers game the system have already been discussed in previous chapters, but my 'favourite' relates to in-utero transfers. Over the decades, the care of these preterm babies has been increasingly centralised into an ever-smaller number of neonatal units and frontline labour ward staff spend many hours contacting these units vying for their mothers to be prioritised over others. Service users are rarely aware of this behind-the-scenes wrangling undertaken on their behalf, but it is a vital part of keeping maternity care safe. To discourage the practice of deflecting incoming referrals, it was agreed that receiving neonatal units were paid more for looking after in-utero transfers compared with 'one of their own'. Within weeks, the message sent to the frontline was 'accept as many as possible even if it means transferring our own out'. This hateful practice of placing women with vulnerable pregnancies in transfer ambulances and forcing them to deliver far from home in a perverse game of exchanging patients between units for extra revenue was discontinued after the unintended consequences were revealed, but it serves as a great example of how warped priorities have contributed to a broken service.

Corruption, cover-ups, coercion and collusion

The 'four Cs' are classic hallmarks of any failing organisation and are not specific to maternity. In 2017, the NHS Counter Fraud Authority (cfa.nhs.uk) was established to identify 'economic crimes' taking place in NHS institutions. In an organisation as vast and poorly administered as the NHS, embezzlement of public funds by those who control the purse strings is not difficult. This organisation estimates that the NHS is vulnerable to £1.316 billion worth of fraud each year.

Independent national inquiries into maternity care often highlight 'lack of transparency', in other words cover-ups, but do not take the trouble to identify the perpetrators. The incentives for under-reporting and downgrading of adverse outcomes have been discussed in Chapter 4, but simpler examples include the 'losing' of CTG recordings from babies who have suffered hypoxic brain damage: classic burying of evidence made harder, but not impossible, by digital documentation.

Like cover-ups, coercion is also the result of misplaced priorities. The best example of this was the impetus to lower the national caesarean rate discussed in Chapter 4. This was marketed as 'giving mothers the natural birthing experience they want', but the financial rewards offered to trusts who achieved 'successful' results provided a strong incentive too. The latter would not necessarily have been known to or mentioned by frontline staff discussing mode of delivery, in particular VBAC, with mothers during appointments at 'birth options' clinics. Interestingly, all the evidence suggests that encouraging VBAC in all women was not cost effective, because the 'savings' made as a result of successful attempts were rapidly offset by the financial losses incurred in funding emergency caesarean sections and the higher risks of complications in the unsuccessful cases (Bick 2004).

Frontline staff grapple daily with the pressures placed upon them to pursue agendas that might be unethical and unfair when played out on the shop floor, but managers are oblivious to these internal conflicts because they rarely look service users in the eye and are never personally challenged when things go wrong. When there are calls for 'transparency', managers inevitably focus on whether the facts of the events were documented and conveyed to the mother, whether all the boxes on the VBAC counselling proforma were ticked, whether the duty of candour form was completed by a consultant after the ensuing uterine rupture, and whether the woman was sent a copy of the SI report. But they never admit how their own distorted priorities might have influenced messaging, decision making or care in advance of the disaster.

Why do the media not seek to find and expose the people responsible for the four Cs? The death of sound investigative journalism when it comes to scrutiny of the NHS, which I will discuss in my final chapter, does not help. But even if we ignore this, pinpointing who and what is to blame is not an easy task. It is often said that the reason the Mafia has never really been defeated is that they have infiltrated every aspect of civic society with a veneer of respectability. They have complex but disorganised hierarchical structures and their methods include the practice of co-opting friends and colleagues, causing division such that people who should be working collaboratively end up fighting like rats in a sack, concealing evidence, silencing witnesses, stopping at nothing to secure convictions, operating within boundaries between legitimate and self-serving interests, promising promotion for some and threatening exclusion and elimination for others. All this while at the same time believing their mission is valid.

Discrimination and paranoia

One of the reasons many choose to pursue a career in NHS healthcare is the unassailable opportunities it affords to work with people from all walks of life, both as patients and as colleagues. The duty to provide care to all, irrespective of age, gender, ethnicity, race, religious beliefs or socioeconomic status is enshrined in the Hippocratic oath, the earliest documented expression of an ethical code of practice in the Western world. NHS teams are as eclectic as the population they serve because the NHS has always attracted staff from far-flung corners, but unfortunately discrimination is rife and experienced by both service users and service providers.

Inequalities in healthcare outcomes across medical specialities are often used as an indirect measure of discrimination against disadvantaged groups in society. The first national review to highlight the extent of the problem and discuss the contributory factors was published in 2010 (Department for International Development 2010). Unfortunately, a decade later, the situation appears to have deteriorated, with socioeconomic, geographic and ethnic differences remaining key determinants of poor health and reduced life expectancy (Institute of Health Equity 2020). In maternity care, reports of concerning behaviours exhibited by frontline staff when caring for ethnic minority mothers cannot be dismissed (NHS Race & Health Observatory 2022; Waters 2022; Iacobucci 2022). This phenomenon itself is difficult to explain for two reasons. First, NHS employees are notably diverse themselves – a recent NHS England survey suggests that two fifths (42 per cent) of doctors, dentists and consultants and nearly a third (29.2 per cent) of nurses, midwives and health visitors are from Black and minority ethnic (BAME) backgrounds (NHS England 2023). Second, many staff feel they are victims of discrimination themselves, not only at the hands of their superiors but also from service users (King's Fund 2015; NHS England 2022; Church 2024).

Like most national organisations, the nine protected characteristics of the NHS are in line with the Equality Act 2010 and include age, disability, marriage and civil partnership, race, religion or belief, sex and sexual orientation, but truthfully the NHS has always struggled with discrimination. Its early days were marred by tales of nurses and doctors brought over from abroad who were given inferior roles in unattractive specialities, often in rural areas. And despite many attempts to project a positive image, the NHS today is still far from a shining example of kaleidoscopic unity. A key strategy has been the appointment in all trusts of 'diversity and inclusion champions', but data suggests this has had a limited impact, with recent surveys suggesting more than 50 per cent of BAME NHS staff continue to report reduced opportunities for career development (Ross 2020). Certainly, there is indirect proof of racism insofar as NHS salaries rise as racial demographics become less diverse. In the past, the very highest echelons of trust board management were reserved for white males (Rimmer 2016), which led to criticisms of the 'snowy white peaks' often seen in the corporate sector. This has prompted the adoption of positive discrimination to redress the balance (NHS England 2024). Time will tell if these actions make a difference. Either way, few would disagree that discrimination is a contentious issue, and we should guard against behaviours that fail to harness talent or that fuel division.

The inverse pyramid

I have explained why many frontline workers conclude that the attractions of even a junior position in management trump frontline work, so individuals adapt and assume behaviours or start acting as if they share the priorities of the senior management team. Any frontline worker who has attended management meetings will know the look – the semi-furrowed brow of faux concern, the slightly cocked head and the agreeable nods as their superiors speak in the language of management. With so many directives to action, the drive to recruit staff into management roles is relentless. Indeed, immediately after appointment junior consultants are regularly bombarded by emails offering them 'leadership training'. One promised 'training in diagnostic leadership', 'learning through conversations that make a difference', 'success in shaping growth across systems', 'experience in examining paradigms to sense check your team's mindset', 'using strength appreciation and diversity to redefine norms' and 'self-awareness and conversation modelling skills'. I have no idea what any of this means, but I do believe that the shift away from frontline work and towards immersion into the world of infinite NHS managerial job opportunities described in Chapter 4 has resulted in an 'inverse pyramid' in which there is a top-heavy layer of service organisers whose primary role is to impose ever more elaborate processes upon an ever-shrinking minority of genuinely clinically active service providers.

Obstetric litigation

In 2023/24, obstetric malpractice claims resulted in a staggering £2.8 billion being paid out in compensation, meaning that annual payouts for poor maternity care now cost roughly the same as the annual NHS maternity budget of around £3 billion per year (NHSR 2024). These sums pale into insignificance when inflationary rises in healthcare costs in cases of personal injury are taken into account, with a recent report suggesting the NHS could be facing payouts of over £27 billion for failings in maternity care since 2019 (NHSR 2025).

In Chapter 7, I discussed how legal redress for service users offers the hope of a genuinely objective and in-depth analysis of their care and financial compensation. I also explained how cash-strapped NHS trusts want to guard against reputational damage, so move quickly towards settlement. But failure to mount a credible defence of frontline staff is not only damaging for the individuals concerned but also acts as a deterrent to others considering a career in the speciality. Furthermore, despite NHSR taking pride in a less adversarial approach and resolving more and more cases (more than 80 per cent at present) without court proceedings (NHSR 2024), I believe that it is not always in the long-term interest of the NHS maternity service to be content even with 'no liability' or 'without prejudice' settlements. The UK law works on precedent, so each settlement relating to a particular matter opens the floodgates to similar cases. Today, claimants' solicitors can easily construct a successful case based on thin evidence of wrongdoing in an increasingly wide range of perfectly well-recognised complications in obstetrics that may occur even when care has been exemplary. The long list of obstetric events now widely regarded as 'indefensible' includes most 'missed' fetal anomalies; any complication following instrumental delivery or the vaginal delivery of breech or twins; third- and fourth-degree tears; vaginal prolapse; shoulder dystocia resulting in brachial plexus injury; Asherman's syndrome and many more. The money paid out comes from premiums paid by NHS trusts to NHS Resolution, which of course is just taxpayers' money via a different route. Like many of my colleagues, I am fearful that the financial burden of obstetric litigation may render the NHS maternity service unsustainable (Yau et al 2020). The situation is truly bleak, made worse by the media warning women to 'think twice' before delivering in maternity units with higher than average compensation settlements (Stearn 2025). Given that lessons have not been learnt through risk management, the silver lining is that this may happen as a result of litigation. Indeed, there are publications that claim to offer us hope (Jha & Power 2022), but regrettably I think these efforts will not help. This is because obstetric risk and litigation risk, while overlapping to a small extent, are quite distinct entities. Take, for instance, intrapartum sepsis and primary postpartum haemorrhage, which are often predictable and thus usually preventable. They remain depressingly common and represent major obstetric risk yet rarely feature in litigation unless associated with neonatal infective enceph- alopathy or hysterectomy. In contrast, severe acute intrapartum fetal hypoxia is relatively rare and sometimes unpredictable but, due to the long-term morbidity associated with cerebral palsy, overrepresented in litigation cases, often resulting in eye-watering financial settlements. If the maternity risk management process was fit for purpose, it could distinguish between obstetric risk and litigation risk and ideally promote practices that mitigate against both. But a barrister's wagging finger telling frontline staff what they should have done differently in his or her client's case will not help at all.

A grave concern of mine is that in recent years, mortality cases have been weaponised to bring about criminal proceedings. These can be filed against trusts by charging the organisation with corporate manslaughter, which at present carries a maximum fine of £20 million. In 2021, East Kent Hospitals University NHS Foundation Trust was fined £733,000 for catastrophic failings in its maternity; and in 2023, Nottingham University Hospitals NHS Trust was ordered to pay a fine of £800,000, which was increased in 2025 to over £1.6 million. Individuals can also be charged with gross negligence manslaughter. If found guilty, there is a maximum sentence of life imprisonment. The situation is so serious that it has prompted a review of government policy (Williams Report 2018), but the trend seems unstoppable. In Chapter 6, I discussed Operation Lincoln in West Mercia, but now anyone in any region of the UK can contact the police and report a member of NHS frontline staff they suspect has committed gross negligence manslaughter. It is difficult to counter the impression that there are criminals working within the Service when the public hears of the pain experienced by families whose loved ones were 'looked after' by the rogues of our profession, but the crushing impact of a criminal investigation for frontline staff should not be underestimated. The fact that it has even come to this represents a woeful state of affairs.

A problematic consequence of litigation is that it results in defensive medicine, which, quite apart from being wasteful, further destroys trust between service users and frontline staff. Unnecessary investigations and inpatient admissions are costly and inconvenient to mothers who may be put off reporting symptoms for fear of being confined unnecessarily. Women are often guilted into accepting interventions 'just in case' minor symptoms turn out to be something more serious. Counselling lacks context because the overwhelming priority becomes not to leave oneself exposed to criticism or litigation. A whole language has developed around this style of practice. For example, women are often described as 'declining' a recommended treatment although, as the lawyers are swift to point out, it is not usually stated why. The word 'tokophobia', meaning fear of labour, is commonly documented as a reason for caesarean section undertaken without a recognised medical concern. This condescending term suggests the mother has an irrational fear of vaginal birth, rather than that she has carefully weighed up the pros and cons and decided caesarean was the most acceptable option for her. Although on the face of it they might appear to be opposite extremes, defensive practice is as damaging to patient care as the obsessive natural birthing narrative. In both, information is delivered without context, using coercive wording designed to guilt mothers into submission and acceptance.

'Ineffective leadership'

This phrase appears recurrently in independent national inquiries, and recent criticisms of 'leadership' teams centre on lack of diversity. It is impossible for any review of public services nowadays not to reference prejudice and social inequalities and, while these concerns are valid, the real problem is far, far simpler – namely that there are no leaders. Sure, the maternity service and wider NHS are awash with managers, but that is not to say that these individuals are leaders. The people the independent national inquiries refer to as 'leaders' are those with fancy titles and a long list of positions they have held under the section entitled 'leadership roles' on their CVs. These individuals are simply taking advantage of a healthcare system which has, since the 1990s, allowed ambitious managers to morph into self-proclaimed 'leaders' and cast themselves in these roles without being qualified, competent, accountable, elected or regulated. It has been a catastrophic failing within the NHS to consider managers and leaders as one and the same because the latter is not simply an experienced or trumped-up version of the former.

Managers are heads of teams, authoritative figures who give instructions and orders, and follow rules and regulations. They chart data; they have designated responsibilities with set goals and objectives. Their job is structured; they promote uniformity focusing on targets and day-to-day matters with short-term objectives. Leaders are a very different species altogether, in many ways the exact opposite. They are hard wired to think creatively and prefer problem solving by engaging the team, brainstorming with colleagues, interrogating processes, reinventing workflows and inspiring others by gently influencing situations to promote confidence, flexibility, innovation and improve services. They believe in soft power, thrive on unpredictability, think strategically and plan constructively for long-term sustainability. Their absence in any organisation all but guarantees failure.

Conclusion

What I have described above is a position from which it will be challenging to recover. But it is not an option to allow poor maternity care to become 'normalised' (Campbell 2024), because pregnancy and childbirth will always remain important events in people's lives, and everyone should feel invested in improving maternity care. Considering how we might go about this is a daunting task, but in the next chapter I will discuss some baby steps that might set us off on the correct path.

9 Hitting the reset button

Introduction

It is undisputed that those who have spearheaded independent national maternity inquiries, admittedly with the help of vast teams, have worked hard to deliver their reports. However, these lead investigators usually come from a distinguished background of NHS management, so they see 'the Service' through the prism of their own biases. Their recommendations, more recently termed immediate and essential actions (IEAs), while well intentioned and widely adopted, have not made a difference because most can be filed in the 'more of the same' category. It is sheer insanity to keep doing the same things over and over and expecting different results.

As I have shown throughout this book, the fundamental problem is that the three main stakeholders have different, often competing and occasionally completely opposing priorities. Misalignment of these priorities has continued to propagate decline and, in my view, genuine and sustained improvements in maternity care will only occur when all three parties agree on a unified set of aims and act with a commonality of purpose. There are no quick or easy fixes, but in this chapter, I outline some pointers.

Speak truthfully to service users

Despite all the troubling anecdotes, it is vital that trust between service users and frontline staff is restored because without this any attempt at improving the maternity service will fail.

Mothers are perfectly able to comprehend contextualised data, and these discussions need to start early in pregnancy, ideally pre-conceptually. Many developed countries have a network of pre-pregnancy counselling clinics to address key issues around smoking, diet, BMI, lifestyle and pre-existing medical conditions. A woman who enters pregnancy slim, fit and healthy tips the balance enormously in her favour.

Many pregnancies and births are thankfully uncomplicated, but there should be free and frank discussions about the risks associated with advanced maternal age, assisted conception, overdue pregnancies, preterm delivery, prolonged labour, operative vaginal delivery or caesarean section. Glib phrases such as 'pelvic floor damage' cover a huge spectrum of problems affecting many women, well over 10 per cent in some studies (Urbankova et al 2019), yet this is rarely discussed in factual terms in patient information leaflets (NHS Inform 2025), so most only find out about this after delivery. Similarly, many term babies, up to one in 12, will develop complications in the neonatal period, which may necessitate admission to a special care unit for investigation and treatment (Bliss 2024), but most parents are not prepared for this eventuality. It is vital that frontline staff feel able to have these conversations with mothers, who in turn must be ready to hear these messages and not bury their heads in the sand. Individuals or organisations that peddle unrealistic pregnancy and birthing narratives should be challenged.

Each individual pregnancy carries a whole spectrum of possible outcomes, thankfully mostly good, even if no care is provided. Our young demographic means that mothers and babies frequently 'bounce back' from precarious situations and make a full recovery, but relying on physiology to correct poor practice is unwise. A functional maternity service is one that is set up to detect potential problems and offer timely intervention to avert disaster. A zero-tolerance approach will sometimes mean that interventions are undertaken 'unnecessarily' but this is often only clear in retrospect. Intervention is not a dirty word. As discussed in Chapter 2, history has taught us that interventions such as the use of uterotonics and antibiotics have saved the lives of millions of pregnant women. Increased intervention does not guarantee a good outcome, but lack of timely intervention places both mother and baby at a disadvantage. In Chapter 4, I highlighted the consequences of the obsessive pursuit to reduce the national caesarean section rate. This shameful policy, which many other countries challenged (Betran et al 2016), never achieved its aim because most women who needed caesarean delivery ultimately got one anyway and, far from declining, the national caesarean rates kept rising steadily. However, many caesareans were done as end-stage interventions, which occurred too late to make a positive difference. Timing is everything in obstetrics and delaying proactive intervention increases risk. The popular counternarrative of 'unnecessary caesarean sections' should also be challenged because all the evidence points to the contrary. None of the 'deep dives' commissioned by maternity service managers to investigate the actions of apparently wayward frontline staff, criticised for their lack of commitment to the edict of lowering the caesarean section rate, showed that these interventions were unnecessary. If anything, reviews into poor maternity care frequently conclude that delivery, most often by caesarean section, should have been expedited earlier.

The message to service users should be loud and clear. If frontline staff offer operative vaginal delivery or caesarean section, it is not because they are a bit bored and have nothing better to do or, as I overheard an antenatal class instructor once tell her expectant parents, 'because the junior doctors need the practice'. It is because they have good grounds to believe such interventions, if undertaken in a timely fashion, will tip the balance in favour of a better outcome. That said, some of the criticisms regarding over-intervention *are* valid and these mostly arise due to clinical inexperience or defensive practice. Finding the right balance requires careful individualised clinical assessment and fear-free communication between service users and service providers.

Reassess priorities for maternity care

I believe it should be made clear to service users that the care that is offered is based on the resources available, even though this represents a false economy when the consequences of less sensitive or limited testing are uncovered. Take Down syndrome screening, which is offered to all pregnant women in the UK. Results are reported as 'low risk' or 'high risk' according to a cut-off agreed by the UK National Screening Committee (UK Government 2024) and alternative, better-performing tests are not discussed because they are typically available only in the private sector. Selective rather than routine screening programmes such as those for gestational diabetes will, by definition, 'miss' disease in some cases, but mothers are frequently told they 'do not need' or 'do not qualify' for these tests. Unlike many developed countries, in the UK, fetal size is assessed using a tape measure, which often fails to detect both small and big babies (Robert et al 2015; Goto 2020), but obstetric scanning is restricted due to the national shortage of sonographers and the need to prioritise scans in earlier gestations. While ultrasound is not perfect, it does perform better than the tape measure, an important consideration given the increased risk of adverse outcome with babies that are significantly smaller or bigger than average. Similarly, screening for Group B haemolytic streptococcus (GBS) is not routinely undertaken in the NHS as it is in other developed countries. GBS can cause neonatal sepsis and rarely, neonatal meningitis, with devastating consequences (Group B Strep Support 2025). In the UK, resources have been prioritised for aspects of care that apparently satisfy client expectation and improve ratings. These include expensive vanity projects such as the installation of birthing pools often used to provide evidence of a service that 'listens and responds to patient feedback'.

Labour and delivery are the most vulnerable times for mother and baby and, without adequate numbers of skilled frontline staff, care during this time will not improve. Induction of labour, a commonly undertaken procedure, is often a stop-start process, and it may feel like an eternity before access to the labour ward finally offers the hope of pain relief or meaningful clinical attention. If the mother spends any time in an area with cubicles or open bays, she and her relatives will see frontline staff lurch from one crisis to another as chaos unfolds. Despite the staunch commitment to dignity and confidentiality that mandatory training preaches to frontline staff, this is impossible to deliver through thin, disposable, health and safety-approved curtains separating them from the outside world, so many 'confidential' conversations are overheard. Frontline staff will try to be pleasant despite being obviously stressed. They will all introduce themselves, but the sheer number means that, as far as the service user is concerned, they will all merge into one.

Once on the labour ward, 'one-to-one care' is unlikely. I have a particular dislike for this phrase simply because it is numerically wrong. As previously discussed, a midwife never looks after one patient; she is in charge of at least two – mother and baby. It is not possible to determine exactly how many mothers do in fact receive so-called 'one-to-one care' based on available data. If the shift is quiet and adequately staffed this may happen but if not, a mother should be prepared to 'share' a midwife with up to three other women. At risk of sounding pithy, this is in reality 'one-to-six care', or 'one-to-seven' if one of the mothers is carrying twins.

In an obstetric emergency, there is likely to be a frantic melee of activity. If she has not been realistically informed of this possibility, it will feel like an assault. If she has, she will feel better able to adjust rapidly from being ignored for hours on end to being a top priority for a short period, before being completely ignored again once the crisis is over. Women frequently describe a sense of abandonment soon after the delivery and to many this feels as if frontline staff do not care, but it is most probably because they have moved on to troubleshoot elsewhere.

Postnatal care has for too long been among the lowest of all funding and staffing priorities and therefore a part of the service that features prominently in patient complaints. However, unlike antenatal and intrapartum care, I believe that issues here are easier to address because not all require frontline midwifery staff. Women frequently describe a lack of uniformed staff, call buzzers going unanswered, being left in soiled bedsheets and delays in administration of pain relief. With the correct training, maternity support workers and nursing associates could shoulder some of these tasks. It should be obvious that breastfeeding support and postnatal physiotherapy, key aspects of postnatal care, cannot be provided by way of patient information leaflets, so investment in lactation specialists and physiotherapists is sorely needed. Slow and inefficient discharge processes need to be streamlined and administrators can be trained to do this so clinical information reaches community midwives and GPs, and ward midwives are freed up to provide direct clinical care.

Crucially, care should not stop once the mother is discharged home. Community midwifery deserves to be supported and championed. Funding for the widespread establishment of 'birth trauma' clinics in response to national independent inquiries has been prioritised in recent years, but perhaps a more positive approach would be to use the postnatal check, which takes place six to eight weeks after delivery, as a forum for concerns to be raised and questions answered for *all* mothers. The aim is to provide good care for everyone, not just to implement reactionary processes when directed to do so after a series of poor outcomes.

Protect and empower frontline staff

There are hardly any problems with NHS maternity care that cannot be addressed by ensuring the availability of adequate numbers of skilled frontline staff, especially midwives (Dahlen et al 2022). These are the actions needed to achieve this:

Identify who they are

It is impossible to improve 'the Service' if the real workers cannot be identified. A simple review of job plans is not good enough. No, this requires pertinent questions to be asked and evidence to back up the answers. Questions such as 'What proportion of your working week is spent in direct contact with a patient?' For clarification, this means physically in the same space as a mother and baby and includes acts such as physical examination, discussion of care options, explanation of laboratory results, performing ultrasound examinations, undertaking procedures or operations. At a push, it might also include attendance at multidisciplinary team meetings. 'When did you last work a weekend shift? Or work on Christmas Day? Or do a shift on a bank holiday?' Again, for the avoidance of doubt, this means physically being present on the shop floor at the start of the designated shift time, wearing a uniform, being in the same space as service users and not leaving until the designated end time of that shift. It does not mean being available for telephone chats with frontline staff in a 'supportive' capacity. Questions such as 'How many babies do you deliver in a week/month/year?' To be clear, this requires one to chart maternal and fetal clinical observations during labour and support the mother as a professionally trained individual is expected to do and, when the time comes, place one's hands on the mother and complete the act of bringing a baby into the world.

Once this is established, remuneration should be prioritised for those providing direct clinical care, with more generous rewards for those with a long history of clinical service, a good track record of attendance and contribution to the out-of-hours service. This should not be controversial, because I hope most people would agree that someone expected to do a highly skilled job, which, by its very nature, impacts enormously on quality of life or at the least on family and social commitments, needs to be incentivised properly.

Return to apprenticeship training

There are major problems with teaching and training in both midwifery and obstetrics. Much of this is the result of reforms, policies, social attitudes, the expectation of a better work–life balance and the adherence to working time directives already discussed, but the contribution made by poor retention of senior staff is not to be underestimated. The phrase 'problems with recruitment and retention' appears everywhere and seems to give equivalence to the two, but retention is by far the more important because it is a precursor to recruitment. Many frontline staff entered specialist training because they were inspired by their predecessors. We all remember people who have shared their wisdom and experience with us or helped shape our careers. Teaching and mentoring matter. Wit, humour and cheeky anecdotes delivered interactively by astute and perceptive trainers, the bedrock of the old-style training programmes, have been replaced by bland, repetitive and mainly online teaching sources that reference the latest guidelines or websites. What has taken over two decades to destroy will, in my view, take at least as long to turn around, but a step in the right direction would be to reintroduce an apprenticeship model of training, which would be made easier by building functional multidisciplinary teams.

Build functional multidisciplinary teams

The 'them and us' way of working has not served us well. Teams need midwives and obstetricians to work together and *not* in parallel as they do in most maternity units at present. Examples of working in parallel include nursing notes or entries being recorded in different files from obstetric notes, meaning clinical concerns or management plans are not shared and can be overlooked or misinterpreted. It is tiresome to complete a ward round then have to find the midwife-in-charge and repeat the clinical care plans, not least of all because some plans will change if the midwife then offers a piece of information that might render the intended care plan inappropriate. Standing shoulder to shoulder on ward rounds saves time, improves communication and ensures care plans are clear. Labour is a particularly vulnerable time and at present, midwives are considered autonomous practitioners for women having uncomplicated births, but they are expected to inform either their seniors or the obstetric team at the first glimpse of something untoward, so the onus is on them to recognise the tipping point. This is not only unnecessarily stressful, but the optics are bad because it feeds into the perception that obstetricians and anaesthetists are only there to intervene when 'things go wrong'. It would be far better to do joint reviews at regular intervals throughout the intrapartum period.

This co-working is not an unknown concept, and many maternity units already have mixed speciality teams working in specific areas, notably for pregnant women with gestational diabetes, where this model has worked well for years. Many units have teams that specialise in the care of women with twins or triplets, or perinatal mental health teams. Others have introduced separately staffed theatre lists for elective caesarean sections. Promoting collaborative working is not rocket science; it's common sense. Realistically, inadequate numbers of frontline staff and modern working time directives will not allow for the medical firm and midwifery team structures of old, but with some creative thinking we could work towards a system of small, stable multidisciplinary teams comprising individuals with a range of experience and skills which would give staff autonomy to practice safety within comfortable but expanding boundaries, knowing they can call upon other members of their team for advice or support – teams in which a genuine sense of camaraderie replaces the selfish individualism and paranoid self-preservation that exists today. The days of moving names around an Excel spreadsheet to fill gaps in rotas and deploying staff randomly in whichever part of the service is deficient on the day must end.

Safeguard psychological wellbeing

Frontline staff should not fear coming to work. It is not wrong for them to expect support, encouragement, rewards and kindness as they go about their everyday tasks. The RCM has issued recommendations on tackling 'poor unit culture', primarily the result of strained relationships between frontline staff and managers, and many units have systems in place that supposedly enable frontline staff to report bullying, harassment or prejudicial behaviour (RCM 2021). In the same way as the mandatory appointment of 'freedom to speak up' champions has not made any tangible difference to the problems faced by NHS whistleblowers, these strategies are unlikely to help frontline maternity staff because they are not naïve enough to raise such concerns in front of individuals most likely to be the perpetrators. Anonymous reporting systems via representatives elected by frontline staff or reporting to an impartial third party outside the trust are steps worth considering.

Aside from the 'in-house' problems, frontline workers are often treated with disrespect by service users. Admittedly, the service can be frustrating and disappointing to its users but nevertheless it is not OK to insult or assault frontline workers. There is no excuse for swearing, spitting, groping or mocking the accents of staff who are working hard in such demanding circumstances. It is not OK to turn up late to clinic and still demand to be seen. It is not OK to have your children run feral around the waiting room, toppling over the water fountain and pulling the cables out of the back of the computers. It is not OK to have your relative film the ultrasound scan despite being asked not to and to insist on asking intrusive questions and demand immediate answers while the sonographer tries to complete a critical assessment of the fetus.

Yet these are daily occurrences, and frontline staff are just expected to accept this; although some units have introduced personal alarms and panic buttons in rooms, most have not. Service users need to understand that it is not the receptionist's fault that the clinic is running late; this is because there are not enough midwives or doctors to see the patients on time. It is not the cleaner's fault that the bins are overflowing, as they have now been allocated to four clinical areas instead of two because there are not enough domestic staff. It is not the porter's fault if a mother has to wait for several hours to be taken to the special care unit to see her baby – they had to bring blood for the blood bank for a haemorrhaging mother and that took priority.

Poor treatment of frontline staff has become acceptable to the extent that only a minority of cases are reported and when they are, it is usually the frontline staff who are questioned and expected to write a report explaining what they did to upset the patient. We must stop stacking the cards against frontline workers and instead offer proper and genuine support by implementing a zero-tolerance approach to staff abuse. This may include escorting abusive relatives off the premises, issuing written warnings, increased hospital security staffing, even police involvement. And crucially, all should be available 24/7 in a speciality where much of the action occurs out of hours.

The task is to create a workplace that is kind and accommodating, demanding yet rewarding, challenging yet supportive. Frontline staff deserve to go home at the end of a shift feeling as though they have done a good job, that they were valued and that they want to return and do the same again tomorrow.

Improve the physical environment

Improving NHS premises is not easy because it requires huge financial investment in large-scale infrastructure projects, but poor working environments do compromise care. I have already discussed the contributors to inefficient workflows, but for frontline staff even small everyday acts can feel uncomfortable, such as calling out a patient's name across a busy waiting area, explaining procedures in a six-bed preoperative bay or performing a vaginal speculum examination behind a fold-away partition. I recall having to counsel a mother about her management options in the sluice room after the sonographer detected spina bifida on the mid-trimester scan. The consultation, during which we were both standing next to a smelly sink, was interrupted by a midwife who attempted to enter carrying a kidney dish containing a freshly delivered placenta. It took only a split second for her to grasp the gravity of the situation, so she turned on her heels and walked away, still holding the placenta. This is hardly a shining example of a service whose spaces are fit for purpose. We should not pretend otherwise. We desperately need clean, quiet and purpose-built spaces where frontline staff can care for pregnant mothers and their babies properly. Both service users and frontline staff deserve this.

The daily fight for basic equipment is exhausting. Frontline staff need tools to do their job well – CTG machines, operating lights that work, an adequate supply of clean scrubs, computers that do not take 15 minutes to log on to, clean bedlinen, regular pharmacy supplies, drip stands and so on. Procurement problems are a constant source of stress. Let's step it up to some real luxuries now – a kettle, microwave or toaster, a coffee room with chairs and a refrigerator that works and is cleaned regularly so that the smell of mould and rancid milk are not features of everyday life; lockers in which to place belongings and shoe shelves to store theatre clogs. NHS hospitals are hotbeds of thieving activity and staff often come to work with minimal possessions, which causes great frustration when extended working hours to cover for insufficient staff are required at short notice. In the past, most hospitals had a staff canteen or doctor's mess, places to rehydrate, eat and chat to colleagues. Ideas on better ways of working, cross-speciality collaborations, amicable resolution of misunderstandings, suggestions of new audit or research projects have all stemmed from conversations conducted in these safe spaces. Quick chats while standing in a queue at the coffee shop surrounded by patients, their relatives and any number of passers-by is a very poor substitute.

Support clinical career progression

Clinically active staff form the backbone of the service, so it is vital that clinical work remains attractive. Flexible working patterns, creche facilities, early and late kids' clubs to cover shift times, grants for study leave or extended role training are all ultimately in the interest of the service user as much as the individual frontliner. As we get older our priorities change: staff with preschool-age children deserve reliable childcare; those with school-age children may want half terms off but might be willing to do extra shifts during term time. Those with older children will not want to take leave during school holidays, and those with elderly relatives may prefer night shifts so they can attend hospital appointments with infirm parents during the day. A service that values its staff recognises this and makes accommodations. Career development should be able to continue throughout these life changes; sometimes accelerated but at other times ambitious plans must be put on the back burner while more pressing domestic or social issues take priority. For too long, frontline staff pursuing non-management careers have been written off, left to stagnate or allowed, even encouraged, to retire early. The maternity service cannot afford to lose them. Why not encourage them to progress into training and mentorship roles, staff management or external review with loyalty bonuses to tempt them? At present managers, many of whom do not understand the machinations of the service, are being paid to do these jobs and they are not being done well.

One of the curious aspects of the modern NHS that causes frontline workers to feel most undervalued is that you are expected to be responsible for providing high-quality and skilled professional care while at the same time being treated like a child. Having to sign a register to prove attendance at training sessions otherwise credit points cannot be claimed is demeaning and, in many cases, illogical, such as the midwife who teaches on the bereavement course being required to attend the annual 'breaking bad news' workshop. Or a consultant colleague who recalls being denied a certificate of attendance for a 'skills and drills' session because he was five minutes late due to a theatre case that overran. I think frontline staff should be treated like the responsible professionals the public expect them to be.

Increase remuneration and rewards for frontline staff

Let's cut to the chase. While it is true that no individual is foolish enough to enter a public service role expecting hefty remuneration or performance-related bonuses, it is not unreasonable to expect salaries to meet the basic cost of living. Just think who you would want in attendance if your partner, wife, girlfriend, sister or friend was getting into trouble during labour. What 'value' do you place on such an individual? Would you expect them to provide care based on a checklist or rely on their many years of experience? Would you expect them to be available at all times of day or night? On weekends or public holidays? And to have access to a supportive team made up of similarly skilled individuals? Until recently, it was considered crass for NHS staff to raise issues about pay. Staff were supposed to provide the service out of the goodness of their hearts and maintain the moral high ground. However, the Covid pandemic and its aftermath made many think again.

Poor remuneration for nurses and midwives has long been recognised. Their salaries have been falling in real terms for two decades and failing to deliver decent, inflation-proof pay awards has caused frustration (RCM 2025), a problem compounded by unpaid overtime mentioned previously, all leading inevitably to the strike action of recent years. The pay scales for doctors are undoubtedly more generous, and in fairness most junior doctors readily admit that they are hardly on the breadline, but they are equally quick to point out that there are very few professions that require such prolonged training and have such a high level of responsibility attached to them yet pay so little. Indeed, their salaries too have been subject to a real term decrease since 2008, prompting ongoing strikes since 2023 and calls for the restorative 30 per cent rise in salaries discussed previously. This is dangerous territory because medicine in the UK is now a predominantly female profession, and some doctors may question whether it is worthwhile juggling family life with thankless professional commitments in later years. At the other end of the NHS pay scale, there are ancillary support staff without whom no aspect of the NHS service functions. Porters, cleaners, canteen staff, maternity support workers and the like who earn barely more than the minimum wage, yet the jobs they do are critical.

Intelligent decisions about remuneration going forward should distinguish between pay for clinical activity versus non-clinical activity because at present when the government announce a 'pay rise for NHS staff', the public needs to understand that many individuals benefiting from this are not working on the frontline.

Get to grips with failing clinical safety strategies

Refocus on hotspots

I have explained how clinical safety strategies have been misappropriated to reduce cost, meet compliance targets, prove to patients that their concerns are being heard and action is being taken, and, as a consequence of all of these, improve trust ratings. This has gone on for so long that everyone has forgotten what clinical safety strategies are really there to do, which is quite simply to identify and address 'hotspots', ie aspects of the service where there is increased risk of harm to patients. Importantly, different units will have different hotspots.

The media has highlighted worse outcomes for patients admitted to NHS facilities at weekends (Freemantle 2015), which prompted the 24/7 service debacle, although there is little evidence this is a hotspot for maternity. However, others exist, such as the care of women running into difficulties at the time of shift handover due to the elaborate and lengthy handover processes required in modern-day obstetric care, which means that for prolonged periods of time skeleton staff are in attendance on the shop floor. An obvious solution is to split the frontline staff into a multidisciplinary 'bridging team' so that half are brought up to speed on potentially complicated patients and available to action time-sensitive care while the rest hand over more routine cases. Better still would be to reduce the number of handovers and, although the 24-hour shifts of old would not be permissible today, certainly a review of the labour ward team timetabling schedule would be in order for many units addressing both the hotspot issue and continuity of care.

Another common hotspot is assessment and management of acute non-labouring admissions. In recognition of this, there is likely to be widespread adoption of the Birmingham Symptom-specific Obstetric Triage System, or BSOTS (RCOG 2023), over the next few years. This system stipulates that mothers are to be assessed within 15 minutes of arrival to a maternity triage area and categorised as green, yellow, orange or red according to the level of concern, with further time-limited actions to follow. I am sceptical as to whether this will improve matters in practice for several reasons, including lack of experienced staff at initial contact, inefficient workflows and the fact that similar classification systems with time-limited actions, such as those relating to CTG monitoring, have not proved their worth. I hope I am wrong.

Re-evaluate evidence-based practice and clinical guidelines

The obsession with evidence-based practice and clinical guidelines keeps drawing us down into the quicksand that is called standardised care. Undoubtedly, there are certain aspects of clinical care (very few) that lend themselves perfectly to being standardised, typically when the diagnosis, patient expectation and aims of treatment are entirely clear, for example neonatal cardiopulmonary resuscitation or the administration of insulin sliding scales for a pregnant woman with diabetes. In most clinical situations, however, the picture is not black or white, and clinical care should be based on an individualised approach in which a composite of multiple strands of case-specific factors is woven together to create a fuller picture. Experienced frontline staff know which aspects of care lend themselves to a standardised approach and which do not and, if allowed to practice intuitively, they will flex between the two without even realising.

This time-honoured approach to clinical care respects a patient's characteristics, acknowledges their wishes and answers their questions based on the care provider's experience and foresight. Anything else is just following an instruction manual. The obsession with 'standardisation' is a bizarre direction of travel, given that in many healthcare systems, there is a thrust to adopt more 'personalised care'. In the NHS this phrase is used to describe care in accordance with the patient choice but in other developed healthcare systems this means something quite different. It relates to the targeting care based on assessment of individual attributes and likely responses – for example, screening programmes adapted to look for disease based on genetic information about an individual's predisposition, use of familial biomarkers and other algorithms. Similarly, pharmaceutical companies are now routinely analysing molecular and cellular data of individuals as a means of predicting therapeutic response.

The maternity service as it exists today is built on mountains of unrealistic guidelines, drop-down auto-populated screens, disclaimers at the end of reports or nonsensical consent forms with slapped-on stickers listing risks and complications to operative procedures. This 'one size fits all' approach repels patients who have a distaste for 'production line' care and leaves frontline staff vulnerable to entirely valid criticisms of failing to address the specifics of the case. The situation has spiralled out of control to the point that, if stripped of these guidelines, some frontline staff feel naked. Improvement will only happen if they relearn how to approach clinical problems thoughtfully and go back to the apprenticeship model of training and mentoring within stable, functional multidisciplinary teams.

Repurpose audit

Large-scale national audits are useful, although the requirement for trusts to provide maternity outcome data to an ever-increasing number of national reporting systems, many of which overlap, is exhausting, and a more streamlined approach would encourage continued engagement. In contrast, local audits need to be redesigned to address local maternity service needs. There should be a clear distinction between data collected for management purposes (maternity benchmarking, CNST or similar financial initiative schemes) and data collected to address shortcomings in care. We must stop labouring under the misapprehension that these are the same. Examples of the latter include: numbers of cancelled elective cases, delays resulting in deteriorating clinical condition, mode of delivery in gestational diabetes according to treatment, induction of labour outcomes according to indication, start to completion times for induced labours, outcomes following prolonged use of oxytocin or prolonged second stage, outcomes for postdates pregnancies, prevalence of meconium-related neonatal problems, complications of second-stage caesarean deliveries, pelvic floor follow-up studies following instrumental deliveries versus spontaneous vaginal deliveries, to list but a few. I mention these because they are hotspots that feature disproportionately in adverse outcomes but are rarely scrutinised because they do not have targets attached to them. Clinical audit can be a powerful tool for improvement if used thoughtfully.

Tackle maternity risk management

This is the bleeding heart of the NHS maternity service. It is difficult to know where to start, but central to addressing this will be recognition that this process must no longer be used for managerial leverage or to play games with the careers of frontline staff. Studies have shown that it is often not the clinical issues or even the difficulties of multitasking that result in harm to patients but rather the stress of working in poorly managed, poorly supported and overdemanding care systems (Gilbert 2025). Thus, any individual who does not participate in daily clinical practice should be removed from this process: it should only be led by experienced clinicians in active practice because only they can distinguish between avoidable and unavoidable adverse harm and interrogate the former in a way that counts. The days of foisting blame on frontline staff and sacrificing individuals when all the evidence points to systemic issues making a vital contribution, such as in the Bawa-Garba case discussed in Chapter 7, must end.

Where there is a combination of factors leading to a poor outcome, the likely relative contribution each makes needs to be determined so that corrective measures are relevant and proportionate. Apportioning responsibility for poor outcomes is not always comfortable territory, so risk management processes have hidden behind the 'no blame' approach, but this has not always served us well. Frontline workers are not naïve; they understand when they have done something wrong and have no interest whatsoever in repeating their mistake. They do, however, deserve a fair crack at discussing mitigating circumstances. They also have the right to have their case heard by people who work at the coalface. In the rare cases where individual failings are clearly responsible, the 'no blame' approach risks alienating the majority of well-performing staff by introducing a host of retraining measures that truthfully only one person needs. The real issues should be addressed discreetly and promptly without irritating co-workers. While individual failings of significant magnitude are mercifully infrequent, an omnipresent threat is inadequate staffing, and this can never be addressed by more training. This requires more frontline staff, not harassment of existing staff.

We need to abolish ludicrous phrases that fail to give context to real-life situations. Although rarely used now, a good example is the phrase 'never event' used to describe, among other things, a retained surgical swab. Of course, this is neither desirable nor intentional, but not once have I heard anyone on a maternity risk management panel challenge this phrase. Perhaps knowledge of the gut-wrenching terror felt as you try to stem a postpartum haemorrhage and save the life of the mother needs to be felt to be understood, but it would be the view of most frontline clinicians that if this loathsome phrase needed to be used any at all it should surely refer to maternal death. The retained swab was unfortunate, but at least she is alive to tell you about it. That is not to say there are no lessons to be learnt: perhaps the haemorrhage should have been managed differently? Or could have been avoided in the first place? Or the swab counting processes after such a tumultuous event need to be tightened? Maybe the patient's recurrent presentations with non-specific abdominal or pelvic pain after her delivery should have been investigated more thoroughly. All of these can and should be addressed, but to call it a 'never event' is quite frankly offensive. Frontline staff try to choose words and language very carefully when discussing issues with service users so as to minimise anxiety, anguish or insult. They do not always get this right, but at least they try. Unfortunately, no attempts have been made to offer frontline staff the same courtesy.

Mistakes and complications in clinical practice happen; this should be an accepted fact. But the patient is not the only victim. Clearly it is crucial that the mother and relatives are communicated with well and cared for appropriately after the event. Historically, the NHS has not always been open and honest with patients, but in 2014 the government introduced a statutory duty of candour for all NHS trusts, which in practice requires a senior member of staff, typically a consultant, to apologise to the patient and reassure them that their case will be thoroughly investigated and the findings shared in due course. This imperfect process rarely placates service users in my experience, but it does serve to acknowledge their plight. However, the second victim is overlooked. The handling and support offered to frontline staff following an adverse outcome is barely considered. They are supposed to submit themselves to being investigated and cooperate fully while at the same time carry on providing care to others as though nothing had happened. Investigations led by co-workers often add to the hurt.

An obvious way forward for the most serious cases is external review, so in theory the HSIB/MNSI approach was on to something, but in practice their panels are stuffed with all the wrong people, so they have made no difference. Nevertheless, I believe with a lot of planning, organisation and genuine collaborative working among frontline staff across different units, this approach is entirely feasible.

In 2024, the NHS introduced the Patient Safety Incident Response Framework (NHS England 2024), which goes some way to achieving frontline staff involvement, supporting the second victim and taking a more holistic view of contributory factors, but there is no requirement for panel members to be clinically active, so the same people will be in charge, and there is no external review element.

Think again about human factors

Any service that is provided by humans as opposed to machines will be variable. In healthcare, both the service provider and the service user are human, so the variation is amplified. The responsibility for adapting behaviours to supposedly improve clinical outcomes cannot unilaterally rest with caregivers, yet this is the impression given during human factors training because there is no mention of how patient behaviours can also influence outcome. Some patients have personality traits, characteristics and behaviours that undoubtedly predispose them to poorer outcomes, but the assumption is that the patient, just like the airline passenger, is only interested in one thing, which is getting to their destination safely, and to achieve this they will comply with whatever directives are issued to them by the service provider. This is nonsense. Let's get real and stop the silly airline analogies. Both the giving and receiving of healthcare represent a series of deeply human exchanges between two fallible parties, neither of which has the luxury of engaging only with unemotional, automated and robotic systems to achieve a simple solitary endpoint. If we are unable to look at human factors in this way, I would suggest not bothering with this training at all.

Stop wasting resources
Admit that good ratings do not mean good care

Good ratings are achieved by complying with directives from healthcare commissioners and healthcare regulators. Good clinical outcomes are reliant on sufficient numbers of motivated, experienced and autonomous frontline practitioners taking ownership of the service they provide. As independent national inquiries have shown, the two are not connected. Sadly, it is my belief that resourcing the former has come at the expense of the latter. Many other public services are subject to regular inspections and ratings, notably in education where Ofsted has been the focus of significant controversy for years. Dissatisfaction with Ofsted reached a peak after the tragic death of Ruth Perry, head teacher at Caversham Primary School in Berkshire, who took her own life after inspectors downgraded her school. Calls to abolish Ofsted and its rating system, which uses the same words as in healthcare, were initially rejected but uncompromising lobbying by the representatives of the 90 per cent of teachers who considered Ofsted not to be a 'reliable and trusted arbiter of standards' finally won the day and this version of the ratings system was scrapped in September 2024 – albeit replaced by an almost indistinguishable alternative.

In healthcare, such a personal tragedy is unlikely because management teams are so vast that the burden of a poor rating is shared by many, but the issues raised about whether inspections and ratings are fit for purpose are the same. For example, most units rated as 'needs improvement' or 'inadequate' have similar morbidity data on haemorrhage, sepsis, third degree tears or admissions to special care units compared with those with 'good' or 'outstanding' ratings. The former were just unlucky that a cluster of cases tipped the balance against them and led to further scrutiny. The tip of the iceberg gets noticed but the great mass of chaos, disorder and danger lurking beneath the surface remains hidden.

Having got over the good rating versus good care hurdle, the next step is to extricate the maternity service from the immoral and vicious cycle of targets, ratings and funding. It is not a coincidence that the two specialities that feature most in the media for all the wrong reasons, namely maternity and A&E, are the two with the most targets. In the summer of 2023, in an uncharacteristically brave move, NHS England scrapped cancer care targets because they had never been met (NHS England 2023). Critics called it an admission of failure, but many on the frontline breathed a sigh of relief. Finally, they could concentrate on the matter in hand, namely providing clinical care to cancer patients, rather than providing compliance data to managers.

Meeting targets has not been shown to improve safety in most medical specialities and maternity is no exception. Many of the units featured in independent maternity inquiries were compliant with CTG and other mandatory training targets, yet their neonatal outcomes were poor. Nationally, the prevalence of hypoxic ischaemic encephalopathy has remained unchanged for decades and, worryingly, the admission rate of term babies to SCBU for low Apgar scores has risen. So, meeting targets in relation to CTG interpretation has achieved nothing. The only thing that will address this problem, which lies at the core of many of the worst outcomes in maternity, is the availability of enough experienced midwives and obstetricians working together on the shop floor, making individual assessments in each case, having a zero-tolerance approach to clinical risk and being able to action interventions promptly with easy access to equipment that works and operating theatres that are fully staffed with equally experienced anaesthetists, surgical scrub teams and competent neonatologists. I defy anyone who feels there is another way to solve the CTG conundrum.

The time has come to choose between good ratings and good care. Choosing the former means things will remain unchanged. Choosing the latter means diverting the vast resources spent on ensuring good ratings towards frontline care.

Dismantle the maternity management apparatus

The first step in dismantling the oppressive and wasteful maternity management apparatus is to interrogate the value any non-clinical activity brings to the service. This *is* controversial because while there will always be a need for some managerial oversight, resources are finite and need to be spent wisely. Healthcare commissioning and healthcare regulation are not wrong in principle, but they have been badly applied in practice. Thus far, I have used numerous uncompli-mentary anecdotes to make certain points, but that is not to say that all maternity managers are egregiously incompetent or self-serving. I have seen some positive examples of patient care being placed first and foremost, and worked alongside managers who know their teams well and act swiftly to protect frontline staff from unfair criticism, abuse or workplace disharmony.

The NHS does not need an insurrection. Frontline workers are hardly gripped with a burning sense of revolutionary zeal. They just want to get on and do their jobs. But the current system does need recalibration so that the progressive hollowing out of the frontline service in favour of management is reversed. Any manager worth their salt will admit that only frontline staff matter when it comes to ploughing through the workload and a manager's role should be about providing support. But managers have been allowed to take centre stage and become the stars of the show, and it is my opinion that the time has come to ask some probing questions, such as:

+ Is it right that so many clinicians are being paid to do non-clinical work?
+ How many targets are not met or abandoned?
+ How long does an average senior manager stay in post?
+ How much managerial work is done remotely?
+ How is it possible to support your workers if you are working from home?
+ What is the sickness rate among managers?
+ Why are improvements not sustained?
+ What is reasonable remuneration for management versus clinical roles?
+ Can the exorbitant salaries of some of the top NHS executives be justified?

Frontline staff are required to demonstrate that their actions and recommendations result in improved patient care albeit according to the utterly imperfect principles of evidence-based practice, yet management processes are never placed under a similar spotlight. And what about certification and professional regulation? Why should this be a requirement for midwives and doctors but not managers? Also, how is the service impacted if managers are absent? There are no answers to any of these questions because NHS managers are treated as sacred cows whose number, existence, purpose or value must never be questioned.

Deliver choice and accountability... for all

In a democratic society, the right to choose is inviolable, but we should have conversations about responsibilities as well as rights.

Independent inquiries increasingly focus on anecdotes in which mothers' concerns are dismissed, their choices disregarded or their requests overturned. These incidents have attracted the sympathy of politicians who, keen to please the electorate, endorse initiatives aimed at empowering clients in shaping the service. But promoting the notion that the service should be redesigned entirely according to the wishes of the service user risks crossing the fine line between patient-centred care and patient-led care. Patient-centred care emphasises the importance of frontline staff making an individualised assessment of each case and, in collaboration with the patient, providing care which focuses on clinical safety. Patient-led care focuses on the patient's individual preferences and prioritises the patient's choice or experience, sometimes at the expense of safety. For example, if the offer of induction of labour on grounds of fetal growth restriction is declined by the mother, then the staff are duty bound to support (not agree with, just support) this choice. But what if the mother attends two days later with an intrauterine death? Or she attends for monitoring and has a pathological CTG resulting in an emergency caesarean section and a baby with cerebral palsy? Who is responsible for that? Discussing the contribution that mothers and their relatives make to poor outcomes is uncomfortable territory for many, but these conversations are vital in order to recalibrate the relationship between service users and service providers in a way that will allow rebuilding the service in the longer term.

I have already discussed how frontline staff are always first in line when blame is apportioned, whereas managers are generally absolved of any personal responsibility due to their strength in number and rapidly changing roles. News of the senior management team at the Shrewsbury and Telford NHS Trust being promoted and well remunerated following the maternity scandal caused much distress among frontline workers and patients (Parket 2022). However, in 2024, following the public outcry in relation to a series of neonatal deaths at the Countess of Chester Hospital, queries arose as to how much managers knew and what actions they had taken to protect patients. A petition calling for NHS managers to be registered and regulated by an independent governing body was started and, although the mission failed to maintain sufficient momentum, this did prompt a public inquiry (the Thirlwall Inquiry) into the wider circumstances surrounding the care of these babies. Among other matters, the inquiry, which is ongoing at the time of writing, will seek to establish whether the conduct and actions of members of the trust board and senior managers as well as frontline staff were appropriate; whether concerns were escalated to external bodies in a timely manner; and whether aspects of the trust's culture, management and governance structures contributed to the failings.

Challenge the broken medicolegal system

It goes without saying that the NHS must reconcile its debt to those afflicted by its failings, but as a society we cannot afford to pay reparations in every case. Complex cases deserve scrutiny, but expert opinions must be fair, balanced *and* realistic. Most expert witnesses are white males aged 50–70 years, often with a long list of publications on their CV and a string of distinguished academic titles. But these individuals do not represent the demographic found sweating with the anxiety and stress of multitasking at 3 am on a heaving labour ward with multiple competing clinical priorities and only three midwives and one anaesthetist at their disposal.

For cases that require 'lived experience', the extent to which these venerated individuals understand the realities of the service and are able to convey its imperfections to their instructing solicitors or barristers is limited. Their suitability for their role as an expert witness has nothing to do with their day-to-day work but rather their command of the English language, their ability to answer questions using the language of the law and their cultural assimilation to those interrogating them. In other words, should the case go to trial, they would 'look the part' and solicitors and barristers take great comfort in this. In contrast, the midwife or registrar being admonished will most likely lack the confidence and eloquence to respond to questions and, in all probability, English may not be their mother tongue. Thus, the primary aim as far as the legal profession is concerned is to avoid court appearances at all costs because barristers, as they are only too keen to keep telling us, 'do not like to lose'.

Thus, it no longer matters whether the guidelines were followed, whether most practitioners would have done the same under the circumstances or whether there was a reasonable case for deviation from standard practice. No, the only thing that matters is whether it is recognised, in retrospect, that something else should have been done and/or what the client and her relatives, in retrospect, feel they should have been told about. Settlements are encouraged in all cases where there is a more than 50 per cent chance of the judgement going in favour of the claimant and, with a media-driven pro-victim, anti-public service slant to most accounts of maternity care, it is difficult to imagine any judge would find in favour of the defendant if any harm has come to either mother or baby.

I have tried, unsuccessfully, to understand how this figure of 50 per cent is determined. With so few cases being heard in front of a judge, there are virtually no denominator data upon which cases can be gauged. In practice, I suspect the bar is set much lower than 50 per cent because minor omissions in clinical care, which exist in most cases and are often unrelated to the final outcome, are taken as proof of a systemically weak maternity service unworthy of its day in court. Most lawyers I encounter are pedantic, fretful and anxious characters. That is what makes them good at their jobs. Unlike clinicians, they are deeply uncomfortable with ambiguity, unpredictability or uncertainty. They love a debate but ultimately distil everything into binary form – good/bad or guilty/innocent. Barristers, regarded by many of my frontline colleagues as overqualified amateur actors, always tell us how much they 'love a fight', but they only fight if they know they will win and are only too happy to walk away when things get a bit tricky. Even the slightest sense of failure causes them to disengage.

Now, just imagine if the same applied in other walks of life, say a first division football team that only agrees to play against teams from far lower divisions so they can guarantee a win and otherwise won't play at all? Or a midwife who is unexpectedly faced with a shoulder dystocia and decides not to try to release it in case she fails? Or an obstetrician who steps away from the operating table at a caesarean section for placenta praevia (a condition where the placenta attaches low in the uterus and can cause significant bleeding) because the mother is haemorrhaging so much that he might just lose her? Such cowardice would be unthinkable. Frontline staff play the game, they fight on, sometimes (most of the time, a fact well worth remembering) they win, sometimes they lose, they pick themselves up, dust themselves down and do it all over again the following day. That's how they roll, and that is what makes them good at their job. Ironically, solicitors, barristers and the judiciary are also public servants just like healthcare staff, so when they decide frontline staff are not worth representing, they are threatening the sustainability of the service and thus, albeit indirectly, ultimately letting the public down, but I doubt many of them see it that way.

A broken maternity service coupled with a broken medical litigation service allows all manner of claims to proceed. And because clinical safety strategies and practices around consent are not fit for purpose, it has been neither possible to protect frontline staff against invalid, opportunistic or vexatious claims nor facilitate prompt settlements for legitimate ones. Concerns about the protracted and biased processes that surround obstetric litigation undoubtedly contribute to problems with recruitment and retention of frontline staff, and the misleading messages that add fuel to this fire must be challenged. I outline the most important of these below.

Recognise that good documentation does not exist

There is no such thing as perfect, or even good enough, documentation and to pretend otherwise is an insult to busy frontline staff. Those who believe good care requires frontline staff to chart a long list of complications for every potential management option have no understanding of the empathy and emotional intelligence required to conduct a meaningful clinical consultation. Discussions are highly nuanced and must be carefully balanced between the provider and the receiver of information. Conversations are charged with anecdote, they often take unexpected twists and turns, and non-verbal communication plays a major part. Studies from general practice suggest that only about 10 per cent of patient–doctor consultations rely on verbal communication (Silverman & Kinnersley 2010). How can the remaining 90 per cent be captured in writing? The answer is, of course, that it can't.

Contemporaneous note keeping is another unachievable aspiration. Most entries into medical records are retrospective and clunky software systems offer a menu of drop-down options which encourage brief entries that are bound to miss case-specific details. Free text is often entered as a 'cut and paste' chunk, making it hard to find the small amount of information truly relevant to clinical management. Defensive writing, much loved by litigation lawyers, is time consuming and risks causing offence or upset especially in the modern age when patients can access their electronic records. In short, 'good documentation' is a figment of the lawyer's imagination, and we need to acknowledge that frontline staff will always fall short of the exacting standards set by the legal profession who would find deficiencies in every entry in medical records even though only the litigation cases get scrutinised.

It's simple – communication between frontline service providers and service users is inherently uncapturable in writing. But there are ways of partially addressing this problem. There have been calls on social media recently for all service users to video interactions with maternity staff. Consenting procedures, deliveries, communications with frontline staff and operative procedures are now routinely captured on service users' phones. But why make this a one-way process that could be subject to editing and selective representation? The solution is obvious – in a hostile work environment, all interactions could be recorded by CCTV and encouraging frontline staff to wear body cameras. Either everything is captured on film, or trust is restored and no one feels the need to film, save for a few discreet snaps of mum cuddling her newborn soon after birth. Unpleasant though it might sound, this would protect both parties and crucially, could lend valuable context to interactions between individuals. Today's service users are a generation who capture every aspect of their lives on their smartphones so this would simply level the playing field. The need for perfect documentation would disappear because one would simply play back the relevant footage. We have cried off this solution for a long time, but the police finally got there with CCTV and bodycams and, although far from perfect, with careful safeguards in place, who is to say it will not work in maternity?

Understand the fallacy of 'fully informed consent'

I have no idea what 'fully informed consent' means because, despite undertaking frontline duties every day for several decades now, I still see clinical presentations, outcomes and complications that are unpredictable. In an acute situation, securing consent is critical, but clinical circumstances may only allow for a five-minute conversation, sometimes less. Quite apart from the impossibility of conveying all possible outcomes and outlining all possible alternatives, 'fully informed consent' is an absurd notion because it assumes that what is said is understood and processed in a factual and logical way devoid of any outside influences by the person tasked with deciding whether to give their consent or not.

While there are ongoing debates about style and content, all communication experts agree that communication takes place on the *receiver's* terms. There is no maternity-specific data, but studies assessing patients' understanding and recall of what they are being asked to consent to are not encouraging (Pietrzykowski & Smilowska 2021), with some studies suggesting that, even when engagement and participation can be planned far in advance of the medical intervention, only 50–75 per cent of patients have a good understanding of their situation (Tam et al 2015). In modern-day practice patients are often given information leaflets or directed to websites to help them understand clinical information, but readability scores vary, with studies suggesting only a small minority can be meaningfully understood by most patients (Lampert et al 2016; Jain 2022).

To complicate matters further, increased risk of litigation means there are ever more elaborate lists of complications that care providers are expected to discuss with patients nowadays. However, there is no requirement to assess a patient's understanding of what is being explained or offered to them. In maternity, clients increasingly co-opt birth partners and relatives in helping to make decisions about their care, but in an acute situation, the mother may not have the time to canvass the views of her usual support network. Why should she trust frontline staff? They provide short conversations with dull content quoting facts and figures delivered in an emotional vacuum. She might wonder if the information is complete. Should she ask for another opinion? Why the rush to decide? Will she come to regret her decision? Will her dithering cause harm to her baby? She looks at her birth partner, but ultimately only her signature on the consent form matters. From that moment onwards, frontline staff are framed as the solitary voice of impending doom and with that comes the belief that they are entirely responsible for any misfortune about to unfold. In the event of a bad outcome, it is always the frontline worker who could have and should have said or done something differently. If only they had done their job properly, if only she had been told she would, naturally, have made different choices. But the truth is that 'fully informed consent', especially in an acute situation, is unrealistic and until this fact is acknowledged frontline staff will continue to be subjected to unfair and irrational criticism.

Consent needs a complete rethink. It is ludicrous to have to obtain written consent in acute obstetric emergencies where the mother has little in the way of alternatives, yet there is no need to discuss consent with a mother who wishes to attempt vaginal birth that is associated, not infrequently, with complications that can cause a range of long-term maternal and neonatal morbidities, many of which, some might argue, are preventable by elective caesarean delivery. Indeed, the most commonly held position after an adverse event involving fetal trauma, hypoxic ischaemic encephalopathy or pelvic floor damage is that a caesarean should have been offered/performed earlier. Increasingly frequent is the retrospective assertion that this had been requested by the mother and her birthing partner either electively or earlier in the course of the labour, but that frontline staff dissuaded her or, worse still, denied her request.

In Chapter 6, I explained that clients' perception of risk is not simply a matter of facts and figures. The same is true for consent because, although possibilities and probabilities are important, it is the consequences of the events that should be the focus. For example, the risk of scar rupture at VBAC is often quoted as one in 100–200, which some may consider rare, but the consequences are potentially catastrophic and include acute hypoxic brain damage for the baby and hysterectomy for the mother. Conversely, the risk of bladder damage at caesarean section for a mother undergoing her first caesarean section electively is around one in 800–1,000, and this almost always appears on consent forms despite it being fixable and invariably with no long-term consequences. Oddly, there is no obligation to discuss urinary stress incontinence or pelvic floor damage following vaginal birth which, as discussed previously, affects up to 10 per cent of women and can cause lifelong issues. In short, labour and vaginal birth should be considered active choices for which consent is given rather than the assumed default position. 'Fully informed' is unrealistic but 'realistically informed' is potentially achievable.

Admit that progressive values do not always mean progress

The NHS was established to allow access to healthcare for all, so tolerance and inclusiveness should be baked into the service. In UK society today, we are encouraged to use kind and inclusive language to demonstrate our commitment to these aspirations and avoid words and phrases that suggest prejudgement, hierarchy, conflict or dogma. In the NHS, these values have led to an obsession with changes in nomenclature to describe organisations and processes in a more palatable way. This is why the NHS Litigation Authority was renamed NHS Resolution, the Health and Safety Investigation Branch became Maternal and Neonatal Significant Investigations; serious incident reporting is now the Safety Incident Response Framework; birth preferences replaced birth plans, and so on. But changes in name have not resulted in better care, because the underlying practices have not changed. Making things sound better does not mean that they are better.

The NHS has sought to prove its commitment to progressive values by mandating staff to attend regular diversity and inclusion training courses, to be mindful of what they say or do and be more aware of how their behaviours may be interpreted by others. However, promoting inclusive values should not trump provision of a functional service; both are important. For example, while there is certainly a need to address the discrepancies in maternity outcomes according to ethnicity, there are many other women who fall into similar risk categories based on other variables.

In some cases, political correctness can even compromise care. For example, assisted conception techniques are now widely available to women in their late forties and beyond because it is considered 'unfair' to restrict treatment to younger women. In principle, this sounds reasonable, but it is impossible to ignore the significant increase in maternity and fetal complications in older mothers, and it would seem equally 'unfair' not to warn them lest we be labelled ageist. At present, many go through pregnancy believing that their risk profiles are the same as a 25-year-old who conceived spontaneously. Other examples relate to counselling of parents when prenatal tests suggest findings associated with significant long-term morbidity. For example, if a fetus is noted to have an absent limb on ultrasound examination, it is now expected that counselling takes place without using the word 'disability' and that a prosthetic limb is described as functionally not too dissimilar to the real thing, which is simply not true. Fear of being accused of racism, ageism or prejudice of any sort can put pressure on frontline staff to convey a rosier picture than reality dictates. There is a fine line between spinning a negative into a positive and offering false hope. Frontline staff are not politicians, so their word should be their bond. Treading on eggshells for fear of contravening the rules of progressive liberalism may have consequences that our patients must live with for the rest of their lives.

The most senseless aspect of this fixation with progressive values is the inability to separate observation from judgement. For example, when a woman is described as obese, non-compliant or ill-informed, these are simply adjectives used to describe observations that can impact negatively on pregnancy outcome. They do not mean the mother cares less for her baby or deserves a lower standard of care – those would be judgements and are quite clearly wrong. In fact, being frank about a mother's characteristics may offer opportunities to improve her care. Similarly, if a trainee is described as inexperienced, this should not be misconstrued as unintelligent or incompetent. It just means more clinical exposure and learning support are required. On the other hand, if a trainee is described as lazy or unmotivated and remains so despite efforts to engage them, then there is a genuine problem that will impact on performance irrespective of their gender, sexuality, race, religion and so on. Observation and judgement are quite distinct entities.

Sometimes the adoption of progressive values requires a whole new language to be introduced. For example, the phrases 'pregnant people' or 'chest-feeding' introduced to be gender neutral, nonbinary and encompass transgender individuals who wish to become parents (Pezaro et al 2023; Crossan et al 2023; NHS Patient information 2025) or the term 'perinatal practitioner' to replace 'midwife'. The duty of frontline workers is to care for all pregnant patients in the best way they can to ensure as successful an outcome as possible. The success of this mission is contingent upon delivering high-quality care across all demographics. Inclusion and fairness should apply to everyone. It is wrong to pick and choose when to apply progressive values and when to disregard them. This card cannot be played both ways because it is impossible to be equal and special at the same time.

For anyone who considers these debates new, I would remind them that historically staff working in obstetrics and gynaecology have never shied away from dealing with topics viewed by society as highly controversial in their time. These include the provision of maternity care to unmarried mothers in the 1950s, the introduction of the contraceptive pill in the 1960s, followed by the raging debates about termination of pregnancy. Similarly, the introduction of assisted reproduction techniques in the 1970s to couples struggling to conceive, then extending this to HIV positive mothers and same-sex couples in the 1980s and 1990s. More recently, we have dealt with surrogacy and uterine transplants. I think I can say with complete confidence that as a speciality we have relished these challenges and look forward to the next lot. The only difference between then and now is the angry and toxic nature of these debates, which seems to be part and parcel of the more polarised nature of modern social discourse.

I believe that the enforced adoption of progressive values has imposed restrictions on our sense of humour, social interactions, counselling of patients and ability to give feedback or respond to complaints. It has led to diminished resilience in society and fuels a blame culture where someone or something else is always responsible for failings, under-performance or making someone 'feel bad'. A worrying consequence is that it deters the educationally and socially privileged from entering public service roles because they feel they will be marked out as people who could not possibly be on board with the concept of social justice. The net effect is devastating because these individuals move into the private or corporate sectors and seek alternatives to public-funded services, thus compounding social inequalities, the very problem progressive values were designed to address.

Identify the 'real' leaders

For years now, maternity service 'leaders' have allowed the primacy of cost control and the protection of trust ratings to dictate service strategy. This has resulted in a plethora of mixed and conflicting messages filtering down to the shop floor. For example, was the directive to reduce the caesarean section rate mainly based on cost reduction or was it 'what women wanted'? How does continuity of care sit alongside multi-site workforce rotation? What is the priority – one-to-one care or access to a second opinion? Standardised or individualised care? Why the 'blame culture' with 'no blame' policies in place? How is 'flattening the hierarchy' compatible with 'encouraging escalation'? What about training versus experience – when is one completed and the other achieved and who determines that? Does it matter anyway if we are all supposed to be 'lifelong learners'? Should we discourage autonomous practice in favour of multidisciplinary care? If service users are encouraged to self-advocate, does the midwifery role in this regard need to be redefined? Helping frontline staff navigate these conflicting messages so they can work effectively and collaboratively is necessary, otherwise we risk continued diminution in standards, ongoing inequality in care and lack of workforce solidarity.

In the previous chapter, I flippantly concluded that the NHS maternity service has no leaders. This is because the individuals widely regarded as 'leaders' do not possess the characteristics of *bona fide* leaders. But there *are* people within the service who do possess these characteristics. Below are just a handful of examples.

The cleaner who realises that the procurement department has ordered the wrong size bin bags, goes to another ward where she knows some of the bins are of that size and 'donates' these in return for a few of the correct bin liners to tide her over until a new order is actioned, even if it risks her being reprimanded for 'messing up the budget' by the lead for procurement.

Or the antenatal clinic sister who asks the maternity support worker who used to work as a phlebotomist to take bloods for time-sensitive Down syndrome screening tests and in return she will check BP readings and dip-test urine samples knowing that the best way to get through the workload is for one to act above her pay grade and the other below.

Or the receptionist who books appointments only between 10 am and 3 pm for a woman whose older child has special needs and attends a day care facility during those times.

Or the two obstetric registrars who do a last-minute swap in shifts because one has a boiler leak in her flat.

Or the consultant who is brave enough to query whether the corrective measures suggested by the lead for risk management were appropriate or proportionate.

Or the sonographer who has a quiet word with her previously very punctual colleague who has been reprimanded by the head of antenatal screening for being late several times in the past two weeks and asks not 'What is wrong with you?' but 'How can I help?'

Or the anaesthetist who insists that the fetal monitoring champion releases the labour ward team from their compulsory weekly CTG training meeting so they can come to theatre immediately and deliver the baby with a prolonged bradycardia, even though he knows he will spend the following week writing a letter of apology following the formal complaint she will raise against him.

Or the senior midwife who reassures the tearful student midwife traumatised by her recent experience of a shoulder dystocia that it is normal to feel stressed, then calmly demonstrates all the manoeuvres needed to release shoulders on a mannequin and concludes by saying, 'You see? Next time it will be easier and the mother will be pleased to have you there, even though I am sure you would rather not be. Now, let's have a cup of tea.'

Yes, that's right. It is the frontline workers, varied and imperfect as they are, who have all the true leadership qualities needed to make the maternity services functional and safe because they have skin in the game. They know what the real priorities are.

Conclusion

In this book I have inevitably focused on the barriers to good care, but the NHS maternity service has countless strengths and assets, which, if deployed thoughtfully, are enablers of good care. Achieving a maternity service that everyone can be proud of needs an honest assessment of why the service underperforms, truthful messaging about what the service user should expect, and the courage to divert resources away from wasteful processes and instead direct them towards improved patient care. For far too long, the principles of healthcare commissioning and healthcare regulation have resulted in carrots being dangled at the noses of service organisers who have in turn been forced to use sticks to get service providers to do what is not necessarily in the interest of service users. In my view, experienced and committed service providers are not only the greatest asset but also the only hope of a countervailing force against the manifest destiny of further decline. It is time to face the ultimate choice. Should the real leaders be liberated and allowed to get on with teaching, training, providing care, tackling obstacles and working alongside service users in a meaningful way to shape a service everyone can be proud of, or should we just keep doing 'more of the same'?

10 What are the lessons from maternity?

Introduction

Ironically, maternity should be the easiest bit of the NHS to get right because our demographic is young, mostly healthy and highly motivated. There are no waiting lists: human gestation is limited by a biological timeline and patients are not reliant on a social care system that is at breaking point to facilitate discharge from hospital. Maternity is also the only speciality where demand is not increasing; the UK birth rate has been declining in recent years although focusing on absolute numbers may be misleading due to case complexity. Because of the disproportionate interest maternity attracts, it is easy to think that this speciality is an extreme example of underperformance, but in the allied speciality of gynaecology, recent reports of women being undermined, disbelieved, underinvestigated and left in unnecessary pain or undiagnosed with serious conditions for years have spawned the phrase 'medical misogyny' (UK Parliament 2024). And unfortunately NHS performance in a range of other medical specialities is lapped by other high-income countries (Papanicolas et al 2019; Commission on the Future of the NHS 2021). This includes the NHS's record on stroke (OECD 2023) and cancer care (Knox 2022), waiting lists for elective surgery (King's Fund 2024a), the increased demand for mental health services (NHS England 2023, 2024) and, infamously, A&E waiting times (ONS 2024), which for the first time have been linked to excess deaths (Royal College of Emergency Medicine 2024).

By way of a concluding chapter, I want to discuss three external groups that have shaped perceptions of UK healthcare to date and have a role in shaping the future – the public, the media and politicians. Although the challenges will be different in different medical specialities, it is just possible that addressing problems meaningfully in maternity may act as a blueprint for addressing problems in the wider NHS, and these final three groups all have a role to play as part of this bigger conversation.

The public

The relationship the British public has with the NHS is complicated. The NHS is often described as a national treasure, and certainly, on the face of it, almost everyone in the UK really does seem to love it. There is hardly anyone who does not subscribe to the belief that everyone is equal in the face of disease, and that treatment and care should not be dependent on any factor other than whether we need it. Commoditisation of the Service is considered morally unacceptable, a corrosion of our national values of respect, dignity, integrity and the rejection of human suffering. These beliefs transcend social class, income bracket, educational attainment, political persuasion and cultural or religious identity.

Overt displays of affection for the NHS are common, such as the Thursday evening applause during the Covid-19 pandemic in 2020–21. Children up and down the country painted rainbows and wrote poems and thank you messages to cheer on NHS workers in troubled times. A million members of the public volunteered to help during the first peak of the pandemic (Butler 2020), and a further ten million helped out their communities during lockdown (Jones 2020). And for anyone cynical enough to think that this was only because crises often provoke undue gratitude towards those seen as our saviours, think back to the homage to the NHS at the opening ceremony of the 2012 London Olympics. Dancers dressed in nursing uniforms, the likes of which are no longer seen in modern healthcare establishments, pushed around barred iron beds with coordination and efficiency alien to any modern-day bed manager, while the crowds cheered wildly in support. In 2018, people celebrated the 70-year anniversary of the establishment of the NHS with glowing pride (BBC 2018), although the post-Covid celebrations of the 75-year anniversary were more muted due to other national concerns such as inflation and the cost of living crisis. Yet if we scratch beneath the surface, there is plenty of evidence that all is not as rosy as one might think.

As discussed in Chapter 7, service users have increasingly taken to filing formal complaints against the NHS. This is probably a reflection of growing public unease, increased expectation and organisational changes that encourage customer feedback. In 2023–24 the NHS received 241,922 formal complaints about care, around 30 per cent of which were upheld (NHS Digital 2024). In 2021, the Health Foundation published the findings of a survey of 2,056 adults in England and reported that while the public were overwhelmingly supportive of the NHS, 61 per cent thought it wasted money and 10 per cent thought the NHS would not survive no matter how much investment it received (The Health Foundation 2021). Public opinion continues to deteriorate and in 2024, the King's Fund survey suggested that only 24 per cent of the public are satisfied with the NHS and only 13 per cent are satisfied with social care (King's Fund 2024b). Increasing numbers of patients who are able to afford it are turning to the private sector for one-off procedures (Barker 2025), and many are now turning to healthcare systems in other countries for some operations and treatments. In 2012, some 200,000 patients sought medical advice abroad mainly to bypass long NHS waiting lists (ONS 2023a).

The overall impression is that the public, while overwhelmingly committed to the NHS ideologically, are increasingly aware of, and unwilling to forgive, lapses in efficiency and deteriorations in standards of care and clinical outcomes. When things go wrong, it is easy to frame victims of poor NHS care as collateral damage of a philosophically sound but cash-strapped state-sponsored experiment on the brink of collapse. Some regard the NHS as a romantic relic of postwar idealism or a socialist construct destined for failure in a world of ruthless individualism and entitlement. Others believe that it has become an incurable weeping sore that nothing short of a scorched earth approach will remedy, and that we should stop papering over the cracks and recreate it in a whole new incarnation. In a recent Policy Exchange Report (Bootle et al 2025) the authors admitted that NHS outcomes were 'decidedly mediocre' and the organisation was 'structured in a way that guarantees permanent crisis', although their proposed solution of changing the way healthcare is funded to a social insurance based model with universal coverage is unlikely to be popular with the public. Thus the NHS, despite its difficulties, will continue to evade extinction.

One of the problems the public face when trying to decide if the NHS is a 'good' service or not relates to the difficulties in establishing exactly what its remit is. For example, we like to give the NHS credit for the reduction in infant mortality, smoking cessation or development of new treatments, but truthfully these are often the result of societal changes or research conducted, at least in part, by privately funded drug companies. Many countries with very different healthcare systems have seen even more dramatic improvements in these areas, so why credit the NHS? At the same time the NHS is often 'blamed' for shortcomings and inequalities in clinical outcomes that are in large part outside its control.

Of course, there are examples where the NHS deserves all the credit it is given, notably past successes in teaching and training once the envy of the world, and an outstanding record on research, innovation and in recent years partnerships with industry. The NHS appears to perform best when the message is simple, the public is largely on board and frontline staff are freed up to undertake their role without distractions or interference. Take, for example, the Covid vaccination programme. Although inevitably imperfect due to the rapidity of the rollout, the message was clear. All eligible people should be offered the vaccine and, by and large, the public wanted this at the time so they could reclaim their freedom. Frontline staff were redeployed to vaccinate the population; private drug companies provided the tools, ie the vaccines; and local authorities provided the spaces by converting churches, sports halls and the like into vaccination centres. Data was collected at a national level via the NHS Covid app, and there was a sole aim, ie to vaccinate every eligible person who consented to this. There were no targets, no 'competition', no requirement to submit compliance data, no 'ratings' of vaccination centres, just pure and simple delivery of healthcare.

I believe the time has come for the public to take a long, hard look at the NHS – not through the rose-tinted spectacles of a lovestruck teenager or indeed with the mindset of a disgruntled user waiting interminably for a hip replacement, but with objectivity and a clear focus on what 'the Service' really needs and, crucially, what it does *not*, in order to perform as it should.

The media

Since its establishment, the NHS has been subject to media scrutiny. Cost pressures; poor access to care, especially in rural areas; variable standards of care, especially in general practice; underinvestment in mental health care; and inadequate staffing in hospital settings have been the subject of news reports for decades. Outbreaks of infection, such as contaminated water sources and drug-resistant hospital 'superbugs' such as methicillin-resistant *Staphylococcus aureus*, vancomycin-resistant enterococci, *Clostridium difficile* and carbapenem-resistant *Klebsiella pneumoniae* regularly make headlines. Several high-profile scandals – including the Alder Hey Children's Hospital pathology scandal, where unauthorised removal, retention and disposal of tissue took place between 1988 and 1995; the Bristol Royal Infirmary paediatric cardiac surgery scandal, in which poor standards of care caused the excess deaths of 34 children between 1991 and 1995; and the investigation into the excessively high mortality rate among patients at the Stafford Hospital in the 2000s, which revealed that many had been left starving, thirsty and in soiled bedlinen, deprived of medication and basic nursing and medical care – have left their mark. More recently, the UK government has agreed to pay compensation to the thousands of victims and relatives of the infected blood scandal following the administration of blood products contaminated with hepatitis B, hepatitis C and HIV, which occurred in the 1970s through to the early 1990s. Reports of mistreatment of elderly patients or patients with learning disabilities or autism in NHS-funded residential care homes continue to make headline news.

Today, every media outlet has healthcare correspondents who are supposedly experts in this field, but the way 'the Service' is represented nowadays appears, in my view, harsh, unfair and in many cases, inaccurate. In a crowded marketplace, catching a reader's attention quickly requires messages to be short and simple. There is no room for meaningful debate or in-depth analysis. Reports generally take on a standard format – a damning report is published, a summary of the results is presented, victims of the shoddy service describe the tragic events, NHS 'leaders' are interviewed, they promise that 'lessons will be learnt' and 'improvements will be made'. Little effort goes into interrogating the source data upon which the report is based: anecdotes are used to make sweeping generalisations about 'the Service', and absolutely no trouble is taken to establish what qualifies the NHS 'leader' chosen for interview to opine on the subject, other than that they have a title that makes them sound like they should know what is happening. These reports are not designed to reveal root causes of the problem, expose gaps in accountability or inform public debate. They are written to project a desired narrative and inflame public opinion.

There are common and recurring words, phrases and themes in the media when reporting on the NHS. For example, typical headlines include, 'the NHS is underfunded' or 'NHS staff shortages reach record high' or 'Labour pledges extra funding to clear backlog of cases on waiting list' or 'Tory plan to privatise NHS revealed' or 'Cancer patients say "enough is enough"'. Almost always, blame is pinned on some media-wary politician who rides out the most recent wave of allegations with platitudes and a carefully scripted list of steps the government has taken to address the issues. Without fail, the shadow health secretary scoffs and sneers at these offerings, promising to do much better when in government.

It's worth examining these words and phrases more closely, starting with that old chestnut – 'underfunding'. It is true that successive governments of all parties have continued to pour taxpayers' money into the NHS. In 1972/3 the NHS budget was £36 billion and in 2022/23 it is £212 billion, an average annual increase of 3.8 per cent. Yet clinical outcomes have stagnated, so it may not be simply a matter of how much money is available but rather where the money is being spent. It is not unusual for weak institutions to respond to failure by increasing legislation and imposing ever more authoritarian chains of command to improve performance. The NHS has done this for several decades, but the problem with this approach is that it risks a spiral of decline in which ever more resources are spent on embellishing systems and processes rather than improving care itself. I have given many examples of this in maternity care, and no doubt similar problems exist elsewhere.

Unfortunately, the media does not give widespread coverage to these dull matters, but the data is there for anyone who cares to look for it. For example, in 2015, an independent review into leadership in the NHS described a service in which the pace of reforms caused such an 'administrative, bureaucratic and regulatory burden' as to be unsustainable. The authors described a service suffering from a 'chronic lack of good leaders' able to apply 'common sense' (Rose Report 2015). In 2020, a DHSC report aimed at identifying areas of excess bureaucracy within NHS services in England was published (DHSC 2020). The report discussed in nebulous terms changing the culture and behaviour of organisations, providing digital support and driving forward meaningful change by revoking bureaucratic paralysis and freeing up frontline staff to care for patients better. It was a word salad in which these woolly notions were debated, but it failed to outline a clear plan for recuperating the wasted resources which lie at the heart of the organisation's failings.

Neither of these reports gained the public recognition they deserved. As if to rub salt in the wounds, in May 2022 the Policy Exchange report on specialist healthcare services reported a doubling in numbers of staff working for NHS England from 7,883 in 2020 to 14,515 in 2022 during the height of the Covid-19 pandemic, where it could be argued that the need for frontline staff was at its greatest (Power et al 2022). This one did receive widespread media coverage but only because it reported that during the same period the number of nurses increased by 7 per cent and hospital doctors by 9 per cent, but crucially that the numbers of GPs had reduced by 1 per cent at the time when there was a public outcry regarding poor access to GP services.

The counterargument presented by NHS 'leaders' was that this did not represent a 'real' increase but was mostly the result of various NHS quangos (I forget which of the many) merging. Even the BMA described this report as 'galling' for frontline staff, none of whose recollections of working through the pandemic included someone shouting, 'Help! Please get me a manager here quickly, this patient is about to arrest!' In short, it is time for journalists to stop banging the 'underfunding' drum and ask where the money *is* going rather than where it is not; if they do, they might conclude that the funding *priorities* that are the problem, not funding per se. In March 2022, following the publication of a national inquiry into failings in maternity care, the secretary of state announced a £127 million boost in finances to help tackle the problems and a further £8 million to keep experienced midwives as mentors for the next generation (NHS England 2022), but similar funding uplifts have been received previously without any demonstrable improvement in outcomes.

Now, turning to the word 'shortage', often used by the media to describe resources in its wider sense, not simply funding. A key resource for the NHS is staff. Journalists do not usually trouble themselves to decipher which type of 'staff'; this is just a random word meaning people employed by the NHS. So, I'll run with this for a while. The NHS is famously the fifth biggest employer in the world. 'The Service' employs an astonishing 1.5 million people, and the social care sector another 1.6 million so in combination similar to the population of Wales. These numbers represent some 7 per cent of the UK population of working age, more if part-time work is considered, and their salaries absorb around 50 per cent of the annual DHSC budget. How can an organisation that employs quite so many people be so 'short staffed'? What are they all doing? Well, many (or most – remember, there is no data) are not in patient-facing roles – just think back to all the NHS-affiliated organisations listed in Chapter 4. So, a more accurate headline might be 'frontline staff shortages reach record high'. A recent *Sunday Times* article reported, 'NHS told to cut spending on doctors and nurses to save £4.5bn' (Lintern 2024), here 'NHS' presumably referring to service organisers whose jobs were seemingly not up for debate.

In economic terms, the word 'shortage' is not represented by a number but instead signifies a mismatch between supply and demand – so even in a magical world where there were adequate numbers of frontline staff, this would be no good if demand simply kept rising at a faster rate. 'Demand', also not just a number, is more complex because it encompasses notions not only of need but also expectation and entitlement. Demand in the NHS is often discussed as the inevitable consequence of an ageing population, which the media reassure us is 'a good thing because people are living longer due to better healthcare'. The reader can decide how much of this is due to good healthcare and how much is due to improvements in the wider society, but in any event healthcare demand does increase with increased life expectancy. However, the reality is that demand is often greatest among the younger demographic suffering from chronic disease which is, at least in part, under their control in a way that ageing is not. Poor diet, alcohol and drug use, sedentary jobs, lack of exercise, strained personal relationships, stressful work environments and fractured communities all play a part in poor physical and mental health, which in turn increases demand. It is estimated that in the UK today, there are 43 million people of working age, 9.2 million (21 per cent) of whom are economically inactive. About a third of those, some 2.8 million people, are too ill to hold down a permanent job (Anderson 2021; ONS 2023b). So worryingly, we now have a population that is living longer but is likely to be sick for much of that time.

Probing the delicate balance between supply and demand raises some uncomfortable issues. For example, demand is often driven by factors such as availability or easy access. A healthcare service that is free at the point of delivery is truthfully also open to abuse and the sheer number of missed appointments in the NHS, roughly 5 per cent for GPs and more than 6 per cent for hospital appointments, is testament to the complacent attitude some patients have towards the Service (NHS England 2019). In 2014, a survey of more than 1,700 patients revealed that one in five admitted to using A&E services for non-emergencies (Triggle 2014) and, given the pressures in primary care, this is set to continue. Misuse of the ambulance service and abuse of paramedics regularly make national headlines (Bramwell 2023). The public need to consider whether this situation is sustainable, although I understand why debating these matters grates awkwardly against the national psyche.

Now for the ongoing privatisation threats. Although private obstetric care is accessed by far fewer than 1 per cent of pregnant women, around 10 per cent of the UK population use private healthcare services in other specialities, mainly to 'jump queues' for elective surgery (Gregory 2022). But private healthcare in the UK is largely restricted to profitable one-off procedures and regardless of the large premiums, members soon realise their healthcare insurance policies often have restrictions and large excesses should they wish to raise a claim. Despite the media hysteria surrounding 'privatisation' of the NHS, there is no magical world in which there are sparkling, clean and endlessly long white corridors flanked with well-equipped consulting rooms, imaging suites, operating theatres, uniformed staff and sufficient capacity to mop up all the NHS's cast-offs – and definitely no alternative for the chronically ill or those needing social care.

That is not to say that various aspects of healthcare have not been or should not be funded differently. Many members of the public already pay for certain aspects of care directly, such as dental treatment, prescriptions and glasses. Pharmaceutical companies often provide the NHS with competitively priced products but are nevertheless turning in a profit. Tendering of contracts is commonplace, and in many settings the private sector provides patient transport, diagnostic services, out-of-hours GP services, paediatric community care and mental healthcare. The NHS spends millions of pounds every year on management consulting firms that assess efficiency, productivity, use of resources and help promote partnerships with profit-making organisations (Sommerlad 2024). The media rarely focus on these non-centrally funded inputs into the NHS, and the assumption is that the public are either unaware of or uninterested in them, or content to overlook them.

The 'enough is enough' or 'fighting back' stories usually describe a group of patients who want more from the NHS than is currently being offered. To those affected, limitations imposed on healthcare, such as rationing knee replacement operations only to patients who have reached their target preoperative BMI or restricting access to assisted conception or gender reassignment treatments, may seem deeply unfair. Many 'fighting back' stories focus on expensive drugs not yet approved by NICE or similar regulatory bodies. Frontline workers often share these frustrations with patients; for example, many in my generation will remember the long, hard-won battle to approve antiviral medication for carriers of the HIV virus – a monumental achievement that society now takes for granted.

As new cancer drugs come onto the market, it is inevitable that patients will feel entitled to treatment with the newest and the best. The media often report harrowing anecdotes of patients forced to suffer unnecessarily but for access to these treatments. It is often claimed that such treatments are widely available in the US or Europe and that patients are 'forced to travel abroad for better care', but minor details such as the different funding arrangements in these other countries are omitted, although they may be alluded to indirectly by noting that the patient and relatives 'had to organise crowdfunding in order to get the treatment they needed'. It is really hard to accept that there will never be enough for everyone to have exactly what they need or want at the taxpayer's expense. Drawing lines in the sand and deciding which services deserve funding and which do not – or more realistically, which are funded at the expense of another – is an unenviable job, but failure to have such difficulties presented to the public via mainstream and social media means the debate just isn't being had.

Politicians

One of the amusing things about being a doctor is that people usually assume we are political animals. Yet my colleagues and I often fall silent at social gatherings when the discussion inevitably turns to the latest raft of policies designed to fix the NHS. Our indifference stems from the fact that it does not matter which government is in power. Yes, that's right, we don't care. Let me explain.

Although the Labour Party is always swift to take full credit for all matters relating to the establishment of the NHS in 1948, an act of cosmic achievement in their view, it was in fact the Liberal chancellor of the exchequer, David Lloyd George, who in 1911 introduced a compulsory insurance scheme for workers, mainly in factory-based jobs requiring manual labour in the industrial heartlands of northern England and Scotland. This was later to become the health insurance element of National Insurance, which still provides a proportion of NHS funding today. In 1919, the Ministry of Health was established to oversee the functioning of medical and public health services, as well as the duties of insurance commissioners. This fledgling attempt at socially funded healthcare was boosted by government funding following the tragic loss of lives during World War Two, which prompted action from politicians of the wartime coalition, enthused with a sense of urgency in addressing the growing demand for a centrally funded healthcare system. In December 1942, Sir William Beveridge, a senior civil servant and reputable social economist of the day, presented his cross-party report 'Social Insurance and Allied Services', which established key principles for a state-funded healthcare system, and in February 1944 Conservative minister for health Henry Willink presented the first of many White Papers outlining the proposal for a National Health Service, ideas that were further developed by Aneurin 'Nye' Bevan, Labour health minister between 1945 and 1951. He proposed taking all hospitals into public ownership and the provision of healthcare on a regional basis.

In July 1946, the National Health Service Act was published and, after ferocious debate in Parliament, the bill was passed some months later – but not before it had been rejected by the Conservatives, led by Winston Churchill, on 21 separate occasions. These historic events doubtlessly play into the enduring narrative that Labour is pro and the Conservatives are anti NHS. In any event, on 5 July 1948, the NHS was created with an official unveiling by Mr Bevan at Park Hospital, subsequently renamed Trafford General Hospital, in the great northern city of Manchester, a fitting location in the industrial heartlands of the UK. The guiding principles were, and still are, that the Service would provide state-funded universal, equitable, comprehensive and high-quality care that would be free at the point of delivery. Like all new organisations, the NHS needed a bit of tweaking to get going, but minor tweaks soon gave way to significant reforms, and the pace of change has accelerated exponentially to the point that NHS reforms are now regarded as an inevitable political addiction.

It is important to remember that the NHS was established primarily to address problems of access to healthcare, spawning the overused possessive pronoun 'our' NHS used by all politicians ever since. Notions of quality followed many years later. In 1945, the public was simply promised free healthcare 'from the cradle to the grave', but only a couple of years later the Labour government introduced charges when the reality of the cost of pharmaceuticals, eyecare and dental treatment became apparent. The Conservative governments of the

1950s to mid-1960s were continuously troubled by the deteriorating state of general practice, cost pressures and staffing problems, prompting the mass migration of healthcare workers from abroad to prop up the Service. The predominantly Labour governments of the late 1960s and 1970s presided over multiple rounds of management restructuring, and this period culminated in widespread public-sector strikes as a result of pay freezes aimed at curbing inflation.

Following this, the Conservative government of the 1980s, famous for privatising all nationalised services, took an uncharacteristically pragmatic hands-off approach to the NHS, largely because Mrs Thatcher was shrewd enough to recognise the potential electoral consequences of any meddling. She did, however, remark on the sheer number of NHS employees, in particular questioning the ratio of managers to clinical staff and commissioned the Griffiths Report to address this. Published in 1983, this report recommended limiting managerial power and replacing it with 'clinical leadership', a philosophy that was sound in principle but backfired because it gave carte blanche to clinicians to all but replace non-clinical managers and expand and embellish their non-patient-facing roles.

By the 1990s, the internal market was taking off, but despite increased 'competition', 'patient choice' and the widespread introduction of 'performance measures', which in turn resulted in mergers and closures aimed at streamlining the Service, patient care did not improve. Nevertheless, the Labour government of the late 1990s to early 2000s not only ran with all these concepts but also introduced payment by results and a whole host of targets aimed at improving productivity. It was Mr Blair's Labour government that turned to the independent sector to help clear the ever-increasing waiting list backlogs, something that the loud anti-privatisation voices choose to forget. Independent treatment centres were set up, and the public finance initiative (PFI) was used to fund capital projects, including the development of several hospitals and acute medical centres. This amounted to an exorbitant debt and effectively saddled future generations with a tax burden for decades to come. Trusts that complied with certain targets were offered foundation status, which allowed them greater control of their budgets but with scant evidence that this led to better care.

The global financial crash of 2008 led to empty government coffers. The incoming coalition government chose to address this by introducing a period of 'austerity' in which all public services had to find 'cost savings', most of which disproportionately affected frontline care. The Conservative government of the 2010s tried to course-correct by offering up the laudable but completely unrealistic seven-day Service and found itself fending off objection from junior doctors in strikes – a pattern of behaviour that was to continue for the next decade. In recognition that 'competition' was not working, they also attempted to rebrand healthcare services by using warmer words like 'integration' and 'collaboration' and to quell public discontent by introducing the 'friends and family test'. Problems related to Brexit soon overshadowed concerns about the NHS, but little did the public know that the Service was soon to be forced into the limelight as never before when the Covid pandemic struck in 2020.

The strapline 'Stay at Home, Protect the NHS, Save Lives' became embedded in the national psyche. The fragmented Conservative government that remained post-Covid tried to re-engage with promises of restoring the public confidence in the NHS, stripping out unnecessary bureaucracy, addressing the nation's mental health and improving social care, none of which materialised. In 2024, the prospective Labour government promised to bring down waiting lists but once in office, GPs threatened to work to rule, strikes continued and the health secretary responded by announcing 'zero tolerance for failure', which would come in the form of new league tables, performance measurement, penalties for failing services and the deployment of 'turnaround teams' into struggling units. The response from frontline staff was lukewarm (Clarke 2024); however, partial redemption could be granted if their quango-busting rhetoric proves to make a material difference to their working lives.

Now, I know that we Brits do love to blame our politicians for just about everything, but I don't believe it is their fault entirely that the NHS is in the state it is in. Politicians introduce reforms based on the information their researchers have provided. But if researchers ask the wrong people the wrong questions, then the answers will also be wrong. Most senior healthcare advisors who wander up and down the corridors of the DHSC exuding power are not familiar with the nitty gritty of NHS service delivery. If the public are serious about having a functional NHS, they need to stop blaming the politicians and civil servants for 'breaking the NHS' and instead demand that those in power listen to the shop-floor workers who really are in the know. Crucially, cross-party agreement is needed on all aspects of NHS reform because this is far too important a public service to be ritually tossed about like a party-political football.

Just in case you think I was going to let politicians off the hook completely, of course there are things they can do and matters for which they must be held to account. The first of these relates to communication. People are bored of hearing politicians thanking the NHS for saving their life on the one hand and recounting stories of how they felt vulnerable and let down on the other (BBC News 2020; Pickles 2024). These stories are designed to make politicians seem at one with the electorate, but they often come across as attention seeking, self-serving or, quite frankly, patronising. Politicians must stop blaming increased waiting lists on strike action because this was a problem long before the strikes took off and it is, in fact, the result of a complex series of overlapping problems. I believe they also need to consider very carefully the language they use in relation to NHS staff recruitment from abroad because they often give the impression that the NHS is so deeply unattractive an organisation to work for that only immigrants would agree to do this. The optics here are dangerous because it risks fuelling racial and sectarian tensions. It also deters home-grown talent and paints a picture of a lowly service run by an army of minimum wage workers providing a shoddy service for those who cannot afford anything better. All political parties are guilty of the 'let's immigrate our way out of the NHS workforce crisis' policy, and it is astonishing that they do not recognise that keeping middle- and upper-income earners engaged with the NHS both ideologically and practically, as workers and users of the NHS, is of critical importance in ensuring its sustainability.

Then there is the imperative to sanction state-funded training in nursing and midwifery because at present student debt is a big deterrent to bright and enthusiastic youngsters who are considering these career options. Politicians must not take these people for fools. The midwives and nurses of tomorrow can see the NHS salary scales and do the maths for themselves; they deserve a financial springboard that is unequivocally in the public interest. Which brings me neatly back to fair remuneration and differential pay scales for clinical and non-clinical activity discussed in Chapter 9. Some non-clinical activity is needed and talented individuals with true leadership qualities will no doubt be worth remunerating well, but it is time to trim the fat so that the NHS can forge ahead meaningfully with the right people at the top of the organisation working alongside the civil service and whichever secretary of state and political party is flavour of the day.

An overhaul of procurement procedures and appropriately resourced IT systems should also be a priority. The huge area of public buildings infrastructure needs urgent attention, not to mention drastic action to address the dire state of social care. I think most people would agree that this is a long enough 'to-do list' to be getting on with. Note that this list does not include the introduction of targets, league tables, penalties or rating systems, but rather tasks that represent non-partisan ideals and big aspirations which need bold decision making with politicians from all parties taking the long view as to what is best for the nation's healthcare.

Conclusion

In 2008, following the global financial crash, US President George W Bush famously declared the international banking system to be 'too big to fail', prompting massive government bailout funds to be thrown at the problem and thus the financial industry was pulled back from the abyss. Arguably, the NHS is not only too big but also too vital a service to fail. The financial markets supposedly crashed due to a lack of regulation and too much risk taking, but the NHS is on the brink of collapse due to *overregulation,* which has focused on processes rather than clinical outcomes. Unless there is a major shift in cultural attitudes towards the NHS, a realistic discussion about what is fundable and what is not, and crucially, frontline workers are placed front and centre of 'the Service' so that the disconnect between power and accountability is addressed, we risk sleepwalking our way into the worst healthcare system of all, namely one in which only the wealthy can afford to buy the attention of a specialist nurse, midwife or doctor. This is the type of healthcare that operates in countries with some of the very worst clinical outcomes.

To end with a maternity care example, it is estimated that in the US, one of the richest countries in the world, about a third of pregnant women receive little or no care (Tanne 2023), so this debate is not about wealth but rather about how nations choose to use resources. Truthfully, there is no perfect healthcare system (Bielecki & Nieszporska 2019), but in theory the model of a taxpayer-funded public service is one of the better ones, and I hope that the central take-home message of this book is that ensuring its survival means challenging poor use of resources, treating it with respect, being realistic about what it can offer, and valuing and caring for those who care for patients. The public are the funders of the Service and deserve to be reassured that the resources they provide are spent wisely, purposefully and solely with the aim of improving their health. No other metric matters.

Glossary

Amniocentesis Procedure that involves a sample of amniotic fluid that surrounds the fetus to be drawn and analysed for genetic disease.

Anaesthetics Branch of medicine devoted to the administration of medication aimed at preventing pain and discomfort.

Antenatal The period between becoming pregnant and birth.

Antibiotics Medication used for the treatment of bacterial infection.

Apgar scores Visual assessment of the newborn which generates a grade according to five clinical features (pulse rate, muscle tone, grimace, appearance, respiratory effort) observed within minutes of birth.

Asherman's syndrome Condition in which scar tissue builds up in the uterus.

BAME Black, Asian and minority ethnic Refers to non-white ethnic groups unrelated to country of origin.

Birth asphyxia Situation in which a newborn does not receive enough oxygen around the time of birth, potentially resulting in organ damage.

BMA British Medical Association Trade union and professional body for doctors and medical students in the UK.

BMI Body mass index Equation using weight and height used to assess whether weight is within a healthy or unhealthy range.

Brachial plexus injury Damage to the network of nerves that control movement and sensation in the arm and hand.

Bradycardia	Condition where the heart rate falls below the expected range, potentially risking poor oxygen supply to organs.
Breech	When the fetal position in the uterus is bottom or feet down instead of head down.
NCEPOD National Confidential Enquiry into Patient Outcome and Death	Originally set up in 1988 to investigate deaths in surgical patients and subsequently rolled out to all specialities.
CEMD Confidential Enquiry into Maternal Deaths	A national programme of investigating maternal deaths in UK and Ireland, a process taken over by MBRRACE-UK in 2012.
CEMM Confidential Enquiry into Maternal Morbidity	Investigations of care of women who have survived severe pregnancy complications covering a range of conditions.
CMACE Centre for Maternal and Child Enquiries	Predecessor of MBRRACE-UK.
CNST Clinical Negligence Scheme for Trusts	Financial incentive scheme in which NHS trusts that comply with certain safety standards pay lower indemnity contributions.
Colostrum	The first milk formed in the breast during pregnancy.
Cerebral palsy	Permanent neurological damage caused by abnormal development or damage to the developing brain. Clinical signs may include poor coordination, imbalance, poor posture, muscular weakness, epilepsy and problems with sensation, vision, hearing or speech.

CPD
Continuing professional development

Maintenance and development of knowledge and skills required to perform effectively in a professional context.

Craniotomy

Surgical procedure in which part of the skull bone is pierced or removed to expose the brain.

CTG Cardiotocograph

Method of external in-utero monitoring of the fetal heart rate and maternal contractions.

CQC Care Quality Commission

An independent regulator and inspector of health and social care services in England. It is an executive non-departmental public body established in 2009.

DHSC
Department of Health and Social Care

One of the largest government departments, it determines strategy, funding and the oversight of health and social care systems through its numerous agencies and public bodies.

EBM Evidence-based medicine

The application of best available research to clinical care.

EBP Evidence-based practice

Similar to EBM but encompasses wider based practices relating to delivery of healthcare.

Eclampsia

A serious pregnancy complication characterised by seizures that occur in pregnancy or the postnatal period as a result of elevated blood pressure.

Encephalo-pathy

Impairment in brain function, which can be caused by a number of factors, including infection, toxins, medication, trauma.

Episiotomy

A surgical incision made to the perineum to facilitate vaginal birth.

Fetus

A baby developing in the uterus prior to birth.

Forceps

Metal instrument comprised of two curved blades used to assist vaginal birth.

GDPR General Data Protection Regulation

European Union law that came into effect in 2018, which governs use of all personal data.

Gestation

The period of time between conception and birth. The length of gestation for humans is 40 weeks.

GMC General Medical Council	Regulatory body that protects patients, improves medical education, and takes action when practitioners standards fall short of good medical practice guidance.
HCC Healthcare Commission	Organisation created in 2004 to assess standards of care provided in NHS; its responsibilities were later taken over by the Care Quality Commission (CQC).
Hydrocephalus	A condition where excessive fluid builds up in the brain.
Hypoxic ischaemic encephalo- pathy	Brain damage caused by a lack of oxygen to the brain before birth, which may result in neurological and developmental problems.
HSIB Healthcare Safety Investigation Branch	Organisation that investigates care in cases where harm has occurred to NHS patients without attributing blame or liability.
Hypertension	Elevated blood pressure.
Hysterectomy	Surgical procedure involving removal of the uterus.
IA Intermittent auscultation	A method of intermittently recording the fetal heart rate in labour for mothers considered at low risk of fetal hypoxia.
Induction of labour	A process by which labour is started using medication or procedures aimed at stimulating uterine activity.
Instrumental vaginal delivery	Application of either a vacuum extraction device or forceps to achieve vaginal birth. This term is used inter- changeably with 'operative vaginal delivery'.
Intrapartum	The period of a pregnancy encompassing labour and delivery.
MBRRACE-UK Mothers and Babies: Reducing Risk through Audits and Confidential Enquiries across the UK	A national collaborative programme aimed at providing information to support safe, equitable, high-quality, patient-centred maternal, newborn and infant care.

Meconium — A dark green/brown thick, sticky substance that represents the first bowel movement of a fetus or newborn. If a fetus opens its bowels before delivery, meconium can cause discolouration of the liquor, which is the amniotic fluid that surrounds the baby.

MNSI Maternity and Newborn Safety Investigations — Predecessor of HSIB.

Morbidity — Word used by epidemiologists to describe illness or disease.

Mortality — Word used by epidemiologists to describe death.

Multigravida/ multipara (multiparous) — A woman in a second or subsequent pregnancy.

NAO National Audit Office — Independent public spending watchdog that audits the accounts of public bodies and provides data and briefings to the Committee of Public Accounts.

Nasogastric tube — A flexible plastic tube inserted through the nose and into the stomach.

NCT National Childbirth Trust — A UK charity that supports parents through pregnancy, birth and early parenthood by providing courses, workshops and local activities.

Neonate — An infant aged between birth and 28 days of age.

Neonatology — Branch of medical practice concerned with the treatment and care of newborn babies.

Neuro-observation — A series of clinical tests and assessments aimed at determining the condition of a patient's nervous system.

NHS LA NHS Litigation Authority — An organisation established in 1995, which managed negligence claims against NHS services in England on behalf of its member organisations.

NHSR NHS Resolution — Previously known as the NHS LA but rebranded in 2017 to reflect the government drive towards early resolution and settlement of cases.

NICE National Institute of Health and Care Excellence — Organisation that provides independent advice on treatments which should be available on the NHS in England based on current best practice.

NMC Nursing and Midwifery Council — Independent regulator for nurses, midwives and nursing associates. This organisation maintains a register of all who are eligible to practice in the UK, and sets standards for education, training, conduct and performance.

O&G Obstetrics and gynaecology — Medical speciality that combines care of women during pregnancy and childbirth (obstetrics) and diagnosis and treatment of conditions related to female reproductive organs (gynaecology).

OECD The Organisation of Economic Co-operation and Development — An intergovernmental organisation with 38 member countries founded in 1961 to stimulate economic progress and world trade.

ONS Office for National Statistics — An independent organisation that collects and publishes statistics related to the economy, population and society at national, regional and local levels.

Operative vaginal delivery — Application of either a vacuum extraction device or forceps to achieve vaginal birth. This term is used interchangeably with 'instrumental vaginal delivery'.

Oxytocin — A hormone that is produced by the pituitary gland, which is located at the base of the brain. The hormone causes the uterus to contract in labour and promotes breast milk release after birth.

Palpation — A physical examination performed by placing hands on the patient to assist in clinical assessment, eg to establish the strength of uterine contractions during labour.

PALS Patient Advice and Liaison Service — A confidential advice and support service that provides patients and their families with a point of contact in the event of concerns or problems with care.

Pathological — A term used to describe deviation from the normal expected behaviour of the body as a result of a disease.

PbR Payment by results · A system of paying NHS healthcare providers a standard tariff for each clinical encounter. Originally introduced in 2003 to reduce waiting lists but then adapted in 2010/11 to reward efficiency. Replaced in 2014 by National Tariff Payment System.

Perinatology · Subspeciality of obstetrics relating to the care of mother and fetus during pregnancy and for a 12-month period after birth.

Perinatal mental health · Umbrella term used to describe the mental health status of a mother during pregnancy and for one year following birth.

Perineal tear · Injury to the vagina and skin between the vagina and anus sustained as a result of childbirth. These are classified as first, second, third and fourth-degree tears depending on the type of soft tissue affected.

Perineum · The area of skin between the vagina and the anus.

Physiological · A term used to describe the normal and expected behaviour of a healthy body.

Postdates · Officially this is defined as a pregnancy that has lasted longer than 42 completed weeks, but in practice the term is used interchangeably with overdue and post term and often applied to a pregnancy that has exceeded 40 weeks of gestation.

Postnatal · The period between giving birth and six weeks after.

Postoperative ileus · A temporary slowing down or stopping of the normal function of the bowel following abdominal or pelvic surgery.

Postpartum · The period of time after giving birth, also referred to as the puerperium.

Pre-eclampsia · A pregnancy complication that usually develops in the third trimester and is characterised by elevated blood pressure with protein in the urine. It can lead to eclampsia.

Primagravida /primapara · A woman who is pregnant for the first time.

Prodrome · An early clinical symptom or sign indicating the onset of a disease or illness.

Puerperium · The six-week period after giving birth.

Pyrexia	Fever or rise in body temperature.
RCM Royal College of Midwives	A national professional organisation and trade union dedicated to serving and supporting the practice of midwifery.
RCOG Royal College of Obstetricians & Gynaecologists	A national organisation that aims to improve healthcare for women by setting standards of training and education for doctors and advocating women's health issues worldwide.
RCT Randomised controlled trial	Method of scientific experiment that assesses the impact of treatments or interventions in a group of subjects against a control group.
Resuscitation	Actions or processes aimed at reviving a seriously ill patient.
SCBU Special Care Baby Unit	An area where newborns who need medical observation and treatment are cared for.
Septicaemia	A condition in which infection enters the bloodstream and has the potential to cause organ damage.
Shoulder dystocia	An obstetric emergency in which the baby's front shoulder gets stuck behind the mother's pubic bone after the delivery of the head.
Teratogen	A substance that can cause birth defects or increase the risk of miscarriage or stillbirth.
Trimester	Term used to describe the three stages of pregnancy, each lasting around 13 weeks.
UNICEF United Nations Children's Fund	International charity providing vaccination, healthcare and nutrition to the world's children.
Ureter	The tube that carries urine from the kidney to the bladder.
Uterotonics	Medication that causes the uterus to contract.
Urinary incontinence	Loss of bladder control resulting in unintentional leakage of urine.
Vaginal speculum	Medical instrument used to examine the cervix and vagina.
Vaginal wall prolapse	Condition describing inferior displacement of pelvic organs due to weakness in the pelvic floor muscles.

VBAC Vaginal birth after caesarean — Term used to describe vaginal birth following previous birth by caesarean section.

Venous thrombo-embolism — Condition in which a blood clot blocks a vein causing pain and swelling.

WHO World Health Organization — United Nations agency based in Switzerland responsible for international public health issues.

Work to rule — An act of following contracted working times only, often used as a soft form of industrial action.

References

Chapter 1

Bagot, M & Patient, D (2020) 'Mums blamed for deaths of their babies in NHS's worst ever hospital maternity scandal'. *The Mirror*, 10 December. URL: mirror.co.uk/news/uk-news/breaking-maternity-services-across-england-23145628

Barry, R (2024) '"Cause for national shame": Damning report released into Britain's maternity care'. ITV News, 20 September. URL: itv.com/news/2024-09-18/action-needed-to-avoid-poor-maternity-care-becoming-normalised-watchdog-warns

Birth Trauma (2024) 'Listen to mums: Ending the postcode lottery on perinatal care'. A report by the All-Party Parliamentary Group on Birth Trauma. URL: theo-clarke.org.uk/sites/www.theo-clarke.org.uk/files/2024-05/Birth%20Trauma%20Inquiry%20Report%20for%20Publication_May13_2024.pdf

Cole, N (2022) 'Families affected by Nottingham maternity failures feel "immense relief" after review gets underway'. ITV News, 11 July. URL: itv.com/news/central/2022-07-11/families-affected-by-nottingham-maternity-failures-relieved-as-review-begins

CQC (2015) 'Shrewsbury and Telford Hospital NHS Trust quality report'. URL: api.cqc.org.uk/public/v1/reports/0826982d-e4d9-48da-bc92-a78c8fc9b933?20210518113404

CQC (2018) 'Inspection report on Maternity Services at Shrewsbury and Telford Hospitals NHS Trust'. URL: cqc.org.uk/news/

releases/cqc-publishes-inspection-report-shrewsbury-telford-hospital-nhs-trust

CQC (2021a) 'Inspection report on Maternity Services at Worcestershire Royal Hospitals'. 19 February URL: api. cqc.org.uk/public/v1/reports/3b961c8f-b840-40ed-bb46-1727e69025f9?20221129062700

CQC (2021b) 'CQC prosecutes East Kent Hospital University Foundation Trust for failures in mother and baby's care'. 18 June. URL: cqc.org.uk/news/releases/cqc-prosecutes-east-kent-hospitals-university-nhs-foundation-trust-failures-mother

CQC (2021c) 'CQC publishes a report on maternity services at the Newham University Hospital'. 17 September. URL: cqc.org.uk/news/releases/cqc-publishes-report-maternity-services-newham-university-hospital

CQC (2022) 'Inspection report on maternity services at Nottingham University Hospital NHS Trust'. May. URL: api. cqc.org.uk/public/v1/reports/ba0917c2-37b9-409a-8ea5-e1606163dcb7?20221128135156

CQC (2024) 'National review of maternity services in England 2022 to 2024'. 19 September. URL: cqc.org.uk/publications/maternity-services-2022-2024

CQC (2025) 'CQC takes action to protect people using maternity and neonatal services at Leeds Teaching Hospitals NHS Trust'. 20 June. URL: cqc.org.uk/press-release/cqc-takes-action-protect-people-using-maternity-and-neonatal-services-leeds-teaching

Hansard (2003) 'UK Parliament – Maternity Services (Ashford And St Peter's Hospitals)' debated 7 May. URL: hansard.parliament. uk/Commons/2003-05-07/debates/dc2cc3b4-6134-4adf-9817-fa352f19af62/MaternityServices(AshfordAndStPeterSHospitals)

HCC (2007) 'Letter from Healthcare Commission to CEO of the Trust'. 18 April. URL: sath.nhs.uk/wp-content/uploads/2017/05/Doc-1-Letter-from-Healthcare-Commission-to-Trust-April-2007. pdf

HCC Report (2006) 'Investigation into 10 maternal deaths at, or following delivery at, Northwick Park Hospital, North West London Hospital NHS Trust, between April 2002 and April 2005'. August. URL: minhalexander.com/wp-content/uploads/2016/09/hcc-northwick-park-_tagged.pdf

Johnson, W (2006) 'Watchdog slams maternity unit after 10 women die'. *The Independent,* 23 August. URL: independent.co.uk/life-style/health-and-families/health-news/watchdog-slams-maternity-unit-after-10-women-die-413056.html

Kirkup, B (2015) 'The report of the Morecambe Bay investigation'. March. URL: assets.publishing.service.gov.uk/media/5a7f3d7240f0b62305b85efb/47487_MBI_Accessible_v0.1.pdf

Lally, M (2022) 'The UK's maternity service is utterly broken'. *Grazia Magazine,* 12 January. URL: graziadaily.co.uk/life/in-the-news/midwife-crisis-uk-maternity-service-not-good-enough

Lawless, J (2022) 'UK maternity scandal review finds 200 avoidable baby deaths'. ABC News, 30 March. URL: apnews.com/article/health-europe-7e34210dfd1ec5301aa4daaf7b53b67a

Macdonald, V (2022) 'Revealed: Dozens of deaths and stillbirths at maternity units cost hospital trust £103m in damages over a decade'. Channel 4 News, 14 January. URL: channel4.com/news/revealed-dozens-of-deaths-and-stillbirths-at-maternity-units-cost-hospital-trust-103m-in-damages-over-decade

Maternity Services Review: The Shrewsbury and Telford Hospital NHS Trust (2013) Telford and Wrekin Clinical Commissioning Group, Shropshire Clinical Commissioning Group. URL: apps.telford.gov.uk/CouncilAndDemocracy/Meetings/Download/MTU5OTY%3D

NHS England (2025) 'National maternity investigation launched to drive improvements'. 23 June. URL: www.gov.uk/government/news/national-maternity-investigation-launched-to-drive-improvements

NHS LA (2014) 'Maternity Clinical Risk Management Standards 2013–14. The Shrewsbury and Telford Hospital NHS Trust. Level 3'.

Ockenden, D (2020) 'Emerging findings and recommendations from the Independent Review of Maternity Services at the Shrewsbury and Telford Hospital NHS Trust'. 10 December. URL: assets. publishing.service.gov.uk/media/5fd20f8be90e076637bb5a24/ Independent_review_of_maternity_services_at_Shrewsbury_and_ Telford_Hospital_NHS_Trust.pdf

Ockenden, D (2022) 'Findings, conclusions and essential actions from the independent review of maternity services at the Shrewsbury and Telford Hospital NHS Trust'. 30 March. URL: ockendenmaternityreview.org.uk/wp-content/uploads/2022/03/ FINAL_INDEPENDENT_MATERNITY_REVIEW_OF_ MATERNITY_SERVICES_REPORT.pdf

PA News Agency (2024) '"Alarming declines" in patient safety as maternity care deteriorates – report'. *Dorset Echo,* 12 December. URL: dorsetecho.co.uk/news/national/24789057.alarming-declines-patient-safety-maternity-care-deteriorates---report

Panorama (2022) 'Maternity scandal: Fighting for the truth'. BBC1, 2 March. URL: bbc.co.uk/programmes/m0014sxq

RCM/RCOG (2019) 'Review of Maternity Services at Cwm Taf University Health Board'. 15–17 January. URL: gov.wales/sites/ default/files/publications/2019-04/review-of-maternity-services-at-cwm-taf-health-board_0.pdf

RCOG (2017) 'Review of Maternity Services at Shrewsbury and Telford Hospitals NHS Trust'.

Roberts, E, Steafel, E & Southworth, P (2022) 'Emerging evidence suggests maternity care failures "happening across the country"'. *The Telegraph,* 31 March. URL: telegraph.co.uk/news/2022/03/30/ fears-maternity-care-failures-could-country-wide

Sissons, R & Ashe, I (2025) 'Hundreds of new families added to maternity review'. BBC News, 1 February. URL: bbc.co.uk/news/ articles/cz0lplkg2lpo

Smith, A & Dixon, A (2007) 'The safety of maternity services in England'. The King's Fund, April. URL: archive.kingsfund.org. uk/concern/published_works/000042216

Spencer, B (2018) 'How poor care in NHS maternity units could be causing 600 preventable stillbirths every year'. *Daily Mail*, 30 July. URL: dailymail.co.uk/news/article-6005431/How-poor-care-NHS-maternity-units-causing-600-preventable-stillbirths-year.html

Summers, H (2021) 'Why is maternity care still failing non-white women?'. *Marie Claire,* 20 April. URL: marieclaire.co.uk/life/health-fitness/maternity-care-still-failing-non-white-women-735467

Chapter 2

Barron, J (2022) 'Crumbling buildings and creaking systems: Does the NHS invest enough in capital?' NHS Confederation, 14 November. URL: nhsconfed.org/articles/crumbling-buildings-and-creaking-systems-nhs-capital-investment

Farr, W (1857) 'Report to the Registrar General on the International Statistical Congress at Vienna'. Royal College of Surgeons of England. URL: archive.org/details/b22349364

Fozzard, K, Kelly, E & Zeyad, I (2024) 'The NHS maintenance backlog: Rising costs and falling investment'. The Health Foundation, 20 December. URL: health.org.uk/reports-and-analysis/analysis/the-nhs-maintenance-backlog-rising-costs-and-falling-investment

Loudon, I (1986) 'Deaths in childbed from the eighteenth century to 1935'. *Medical History* 30:1-41. URL: pmc.ncbi.nlm.nih.gov/articles/PMC1139579/pdf/medhist00072-0005.pdf

MBRRACE-UK (2025) 'Maternal mortality 2021–2023'. January. URL: npeu.ox.ac.uk/mbrrace-uk/data-brief/maternal-mortality-2021-2023

OECD (2023) 'Health at a glance 2023: Maternity indicators'. 7 November. URL: oecd.org/en/publications/2023/11/health-at-a-glance-2023_e04f8239.html

ONS (2025a) 'Births in England and Wales: 2024'. URL: ons.gov.uk/peoplepopulationandcommunity/birthsdeathsandmarriages/livebirths/bulletins/birthsummarytablesenglandandwales/2024

ONS (2025b) 'Child and infant mortality in England and Wales: 2023'. URL: ons.gov.uk/peoplepopulationandcommunity/ birthsdeathsandmarriages/deaths/bulletins/childhoodinfantand perinatalmortalityinenglandandwales/2023

Rosling, H & Rönnlund, A R (2018) *Factfulness*. Flatiron Books.

Save the Children (2013) 'State of the world's mothers annual report'. URL: resourcecentre.savethechildren.net/pdf/sowm-full-report_2013.pdf

WHO (2024) 'Adolescent and young adult health'. 26 November. URL: who.int/news-room/fact-sheets/detail/adolescents-health-risks-and-solutions

WHO (2025) 'Maternal mortality'. 7 April. URL: who.int/ news-room/fact-sheets/detail/maternal-mortality

Chapter 3

Bona, S (2023) 'Numberjacks: New calculations reveal growing midwife shortage'. RCM, 5 April. URL: pre.rcm.org.uk/ news-views/rcm-opinion/2023/numberjacks-new-calculations-reveal-growing-midwife-shortage

Elbadrawy, M, Majoko, F & Gasson, J (2008) 'Impact of Calman system and recent reforms of surgical training in gynaecology'. *Journal of Obstetrics and Gynaecology* 28(5):474–7. URL: pubmed.ncbi.nlm.nih.gov/18850417

Galvin, D, O'Reilly, B et al (2023) 'A national survey of surgical training in gynaecology: 2014–2021'. *European Journal of Obstetrics and Gynaecology and Reproductive Biology* 288:135–141. URL: sciencedirect.com/science/article/abs/pii/ S0301211523002968

HMSO (1993) 'Hospital doctors: Training for the future. The report of the working party on specialist medical training'. April. URL: archive.org/details/op1279411-1001

Maternity Incentive Scheme (2025) URL: resolution.nhs.uk/services/ claims-management/clinical-schemes/clinical-negligence-scheme-for-trusts/maternity-incentive-scheme

Newitt, S, Patel, D & McGloin, S (2024) 'Following compassion'. The King's Fund, 29 January. URL: kingsfund.org.uk/insight-and-analysis/blogs/following-compassion

NHS Digital (2023) 'NHS maternity statistics, England, 2022–23'. URL: digital.nhs.uk/data-and-information/publications/statistical/nhs-maternity-statistics/2022-23/deliveries---2023

NHS Digital (2025) 'NHS sickness absence rates'. 30 January. URL: digital.nhs.uk/data-and-information/publications/statistical/nhs-sickness-absence-rates

Penna, D (2024) 'NHS nurses and midwives are "increasingly inexperienced", experts have warned after fears that the recruitment crisis could hamper health service reform'. *The Telegraph,* 2 December. URL:telegraph.co.uk/news/2024/12/02/nhs-nurses-midwives-increasingly-inexperienced-experts-warn

RCM (2015) 'Spending on agency midwives in England'. URL: pre.rcm.org.uk/media/2371/rcm-report-spending-on-agency-midwives-in-england.pdf

RCM (2020) 'Seven out of 10 midwives experience abuse from women and partners during pandemic'. 20 November. URL: pre.rcm.org.uk/media-releases/2020/november/seven-out-of-10-midwives-experience-abuse-from-women-and-partners-during-pandemic-says-rcm

RCM (2021) 'RCM warns of midwife exodus as maternity staffing crisis grows'. 4 October. URL: pre.rcm.org.uk/media-releases/2021/september/rcm-warns-of-midwife-exodus-as-maternity-staffing-crisis-grows

RCOG (2020) 'Later career and retirement report'. URL: rcog.org.uk/media/me2n4tms/later-career-retirement-report.pdf

RCOG (2022) 'RCOG workforce report'. URL: rcog.org.uk/media/wuobyggr/rcog-workforce-report-2022.pdf

Richmond, D & Sherwin, R (2021) 'Maternity and gynaecology: GIRFT Programme national specialty report'. September. URL: gettingitrightfirsttime.co.uk/wp-content/uploads/2021/09/Maternity-and-Gynae-Sept21L.pdf

The UK WHELM study (2018) 'Work, health and emotional lives of midwives in the United Kingdom'. Cardiff University School of Healthcare Sciences. URL: rcm.org.uk/wp-content/uploads/2024/06/work-health-and-emotional-lives-of-midwives-in-the-united-kingdom-the-uk-whelm-study.pdf

Turner, L, Ball, J et al (2024) 'The association between midwifery staffing and reported harmful incidents: A cross-sectional analysis of routinely collected data'. *BMC Health Service Research* 28;24(1):391. URL: pubmed.ncbi.nlm.nih.gov/38549131

UK Central Council (1986) 'Project 2000: A new preparation for practice'. URL: archive.org/details/project2000ukccn0000unit

Chapter 4

Ahmadzia, H K, Grotegut, C A & James, A H (2020) 'A national update on rates of postpartum haemorrhage and related interventions'. *Blood Transfusion,* July 18(4) 247–253. URL: pmc.ncbi.nlm.nih.gov/articles/PMC7375891

Baldwin, J, Brodrick, A et al (2010) 'An innovative toolkit to support normal birth'. *Journal of Midwifery and Women's Health.* 55(3) 270–2. URL: onlinelibrary.wiley.com/doi/epdf/10.1016/j.jmwh.2009.11.013

Black, M, Entwistle, V A et al (2016) 'Vaginal birth after caesarean section: Why is the uptake so low? Insights from a meta-ethnographic synthesis of women's accounts of their birth choices'. *BMJ Open* 6 1–13. URL: pmc.ncbi.nlm.nih.gov/articles/PMC4716170/pdf/bmjopen-2015-008881.pdf

CHKS (Capita Health and Wellbeing Ltd) (2014) 'The quality of clinical coding in the NHS'. September. URL: chks.co.uk/userfiles/files/The_quality_of_clinical_coding_in_the_NHS.pdf

Cody, L (2004) 'Lying and dying in Georgian London's lying-in hospitals'. *Bulletin of Historical Medicine* 78 309–348. URL: jstor.org/stable/44448006

Darzi (2024) 'Independent investigation of the NHS in England'. September. URL: www.gov.uk/government/publications/independent-investigation-of-the-nhs-in-england

Department of Health (2013) 'A simple guide to payment by results in the NHS'. URL: assets.publishing.service.gov.uk/media/5a7c6875e5274a5590059a9f/PbR-Simple-Guide-FINAL.pdf

DHSC (2015) 'New ambition to halve rate of stillbirths and infant deaths'. 13 November. URL: www.gov.uk/government/news/new-ambition-to-halve-rate-of-stillbirths-and-infant-deaths

Duffy, P (2019) *Whistle in the Wind: Life, death, detriment and dismissal in the NHS: A whistleblower's story*. Independently published.

Duffy, P (2021) *Smoke and Mirrors: An NHS whistleblower witch-hunt*. Independently published.

England, J (2020) *NHS Dirty Secrets: Bullying, cover-ups, discrimination, favouritism, whistleblowing*. Independently published.

Gammie, J (2016) 'New ratings show 75% of CCGs failing on maternity care'. *Nursing Times*, 28 October. URL: nursingtimes.net/policies-and-guidance/new-ratings-show-75-of-ccgs-failing-on-maternity-care-28-10-2016

Griffiths Report (1983) 'NHS management inquiry'. The Healthcare Foundation, 6 October. URL: navigator.health.org.uk/theme/griffiths-report-management-nhs

Kirkpatrick, I & Malby, B (2022) 'Is the NHS overmanaged? An in-depth look at one of the most persistent questions on NHS management'. NHS Confederation, 24 January. URL: nhsconfed.org/long-reads/nhs-overmanaged

Lewis, R, Alvarez-Rosete A & Mays, N (2006) 'How to regulate health care in England?' The King's Fund. URL: assets.kingsfund.org.uk/f/256914/x/ee5d760fb3/how_regulate_health_care_england_november_2006.pdf

Mannion, R & Davies, H (2018) 'Understanding organisational culture for healthcare quality improvement'. *BMJ* 363 k4907. URL: bmj.com/content/bmj/363/bmj.k4907.full.pdf

Maternity Care Working Party (2007) 'Making normal birth a reality: Consensus statement from the Maternity Care Working Party'. URL: bhpelopartonormal.pbh.gov.br/estudos_cientificos/arquivos/normal_birth_consensus.pdf

National Maternity Review (2016) 'Better births – improving outcomes of maternity services in England: A five year forward view for maternity care'. URL: england.nhs.uk/wp-content/uploads/2016/02/national-maternity-review-report.pdf

NHS Confederation (2025) 'Abolishing NHS England: What you need to know'. 13 March. URL: nhsconfed.org/publications/abolishing-nhs-england-what-you-need-know

NHS England (2016) Maternity Transformations Programme. URL: www.england.nhs.uk/mat-transformation

NHS England (2017a) 'Managing conflicts of interest: Model policy content for organisations'. 4 April. URL: england.nhs.uk/publication/managing-conflicts-of-interest-model-policy-content-for-organisations

NHS England (2017b) 'New scheme launched to help NHS whistleblowers'. 21 August. URL: england.nhs.uk/2017/08/nhs-whistleblowers-scheme

NHS Institute for Innovation and Improvement (2005) 'Improvement leaders' guide: Leading improvement – personal and organisational development'. URL: england.nhs.uk/improvement-hub/wp-content/uploads/sites/44/2017/11/ILG-3.4-Leading-Improvement.pdf

NHSR (2025) 'Maternity incentive scheme'. URL: resolution.nhs.uk/services/claims-management/clinical-schemes/clinical-negligence-scheme-for-trusts/maternity-incentive-scheme

O'Dowd, A (2010) 'Coding errors in NHS cause up to £1bn worth of inaccurate payments'. *BMJ* 341 4734. URL: bmj.com/content/341/bmj.c4734

Ockenden, D (2022) – see Chapter 1.

Oikonomou, E, Carthey, J et al (2019) 'Patient safety regulation in the NHS: Mapping the regulatory landscape of healthcare'. *BMJ Open* 9 e028663. URL: bmjopen.bmj.com/content/bmjopen/9/7/e028663.full.pdf

Romano, A M & Lothian, J A (2008) 'Promoting, protecting, and supporting normal birth: A look at the evidence'. *Journal of Obstetrics and Gynecological Neonatal Nursing* 37(1) 94–104. URL: pubmed.ncbi.nlm.nih.gov/18226163

The King's Fund (2010) 'The changing role of managers in the NHS'. 14 October. URL: kingsfund.org.uk/insight-and-analysis/articles/changing-role-managers-nhs

The King's Fund (2024) 'Key facts and figures about the NHS'. URL: kingsfund.org.uk/insight-and-analysis/data-and-charts/key-facts-figures-nhs

Townsend, E (2024) 'Hundreds of mothers diverted while in labour'. *Health Services Journal,* 17 December. URL: hsj.co.uk/patient-safety/exclusive-hundreds-of-mothers-diverted-while-in-labour/7038261.article

UK Health Security Agency (2022) 'Vaccine uptake among pregnant women increasing but inequalities persist'. 13 May. URL: www.gov.uk/government/news/vaccine-uptake-among-pregnant-women-increasing-but-inequalities-persist

Walshe, K (2002) 'The rise of regulation in the NHS'. *BMJ* 324(7343) 967–70. URL: pmc.ncbi.nlm.nih.gov/articles/PMC1122908/pdf/967.pdf

Wenzel, L, Robertson, R & Wickens, C (2023) 'What is commissioning and how is it changing'. The King's Fund, 23 July. URL: kingsfund.org.uk/insight-and-analysis/long-reads/what-commissioning-and-how-it-changing

WHO (1985) 'Appropriate technology for birth'. *Lancet* 326 436–437. URL: thelancet.com/journals/lancet/article/PIIS0140-6736(85)92750-3/fulltext

Chapter 5

Alfirevic, Z, Gyte, G M et al (2017) 'Continuous cardiotocography (CTG) as a form of electronic fetal monitoring (EFM) for fetal assessment during labour'. *Cochrane Database Systematic Review,* 3 February. 2017(2) CD006066. URL: ncbi.nlm.nih.gov/articles/PMC6464257/pdf/pmc

DHSC (2015) 'NHS 7-day Services'. 24 July. URL: www.gov.uk/government/collections/nhs-7-day services

Greenhalgh, T, Howick, J & Maskrey, N (2014) 'Evidence based medicine: A movement in crisis?'. *BMJ* 348 3725. URL: bmj.com/content/348/bmj.g3725

Henderson, J, Kurinczuk, J J & Knight, M (2017) 'Resident consultant obstetrician presence on the labour ward versus other models of consultant cover: A systematic review of intrapartum outcomes'. *BJOG* 124(9) 1311–1320. URL: pmc.ncbi.nlm.nih.gov/articles/PMC5574016/pdf/BJO-124-1311.pdf

Kapur, N, Parand, A et al (2015) 'Aviation and healthcare: A comparative review with implications for patient safety'. *Journal of the Royal Society of Medicine* 7(1) 1–10. URL: pmc.ncbi.nlm.nih.gov/articles/PMC4710114/pdf/10.1177_2054270415616548.pdf

Kirkup, B (2015) – see Chapter 1.

Martin, C (2024) 'Out of date IT systems leaves NHS at risk of further cyber attacks'. *Evening Standard,* 8 July. URL: standard.co.uk/news/health/national-cyber-security-centre-london-hospital-ransomware-bbc-b1169298.html

NHS Employers (2025) 'People performance management toolkit: Make time to talk about all aspects of performance'. February. URL: nhsemployers.org/toolkits/people-performance-management-toolkit

NHS England (2013) 'The NHS friends and family test: Guidance for maternity services'. May. URL: england.nhs.uk/wp-content/uploads/2013/09/fft-mat-guide.pdf

NHS England (2019) 'Improving patient safety by introducing a daily Emergency Call Safety Huddle'. 7 February. URL: england.nhs.uk/atlas_case_study/improving-patient-safety-by-introducing-a-daily-emergency-call-safety-huddle

NHS LA (2001) 'Clinical negligence scheme for trusts: Membership rules'. April. URL: resolution.nhs.uk/wp-content/uploads/2018/09/CNST-Rules.pdf

NICE guideline (2022) [NG229] 'Fetal monitoring in labour'. 14 December URL: nice.org.uk/guidance/ng229/chapter/Recommendations

Ockenden, D (2020) – see Chapter 1.

Ockenden, D (2022) – see Chapter 1.

RCOG (2015) 'Each baby counts'. October. URL: rcog.org.uk/media/3fopwy41/each-baby-counts-2015-full-report.pdf

RCOG (2020) 'Assisted vaginal birth – Green-top Guideline No 26'. URL: obgyn.onlinelibrary.wiley.com/doi/epdf/10.1111/1471-0528.16092

RCOG (2022) 'Planned caesarean birth – consent advice No 14'. URL: rcog.org.uk/media/33cnfvs0/planned-caesarean-birth-consent-advice-no-14.pdf

Richmond, D & Sherwin, R (2021) – see Chapter 3.

Scally, G & Donaldson, L J (1998) 'Clinical governance and the drive for quality improvement in the new NHS in England'. *BMJ* 317 61–65. URL: pmc.ncbi.nlm.nih.gov/articles/PMC1113460

Smith, A & Dixon, A (2007) – see Chapter 1.

UK Parliament (2021) '"Blame culture" in maternity safety failures prevents lessons being learnt, says committee'. 6 July. URL: committees.parliament.uk/committee/81/health-and-social-care-committee/news/156351/blame-culture-in-maternity-safety-failures-prevents-lessons-being-learnt-says-committee

Chapter 6

Adams, S (2020) 'One in 20 labour ward mothers are "health tourists": Figures from NHS's biggest hospital trust are a clue to the real cost of maternity care for visitors'. *Daily Mail,* 2 March. URL: dailymail.co.uk/news/article-8060765/One-20-labour-ward-mothers-health-tourists

Birth Trauma (2024) – see Chapter 1.

Care Opinion (2017) 'Midwives are rude, snappy, bossy and impatient'. URL: careopinion.org.uk/346230

Church E (2023) 'Martha's rule: What a new second opinion law will mean for nurses'. *Nursing Times*, 18 September. URL: nursingtimes.net/policies-and-guidance/marthas-rule-how-nurses-involved-18-09-2023

CQC (2024) 'Maternity survey 2024'. 28 November. URL: cqc.org.uk/publications/surveys/maternity-survey

Glaser, E (2021) *Motherhood: A manifesto.* Fourth Estate Publishing.

Glosswitch (2016) 'Birth wars: The politics of childbirth'. *New Statesman,* 17 May. URL: newstatesman.com/politics/2016/05/birth-wars-politics-childbirth

Hayward, E (2023) 'NHS maternity crisis leaves quarter of women helpless'. *The Times,* 11 May. URL: thetimes.com/article/one-in-four-women-left-alone-without-help-while-giving-birth-nhs-maternity-report-vxjh88sxd

Hollowell, J, Rowe, R et al (2015) 'Birthplace in England national prospective cohort study: Further analyses to enhance policy and service delivery decision-making for planned place of birth'. National Institute for Care Research, August 3 36. URL: evidence.nihr.ac.uk/alert/birthplace-in-england-follow-up-analysis-reveals-some-variation-between-units-delivering-maternity-care

Humble, M (1995) 'Women's perspectives on reproductive health and rights. Overview'. *Planned Parenthood Challenges* 2 26–31. URL: pubmed.ncbi.nlm.nih.gov/12346476

MBRRACE-UK (2025) – see Chapter 2.

Mills, M (2023) 'Martha's rule: A hospital escalation system to save patients' lives'. *BMJ*, 9 October. 383:2319. URL: bmj.com/content/383/bmj.p2319

Moujaes, M, & Verrier, D (2021) 'Instagram use, Instamums, and anxiety in mothers of young children'. *Journal of Media Psychology* 33(2) 72–81. URL: doi.org/10.1027/1864-1105/a000282

Murray, J (2024) 'Pregnant women suffer racist and discriminatory abuse at NHS trust, says inquiry head'. *The Guardian*, 24 July. URL: theguardian.com/society/article/2024/jul/24/pregnant-women-suffer-racist-and-discriminatory-abuse-at-nhs-trust-says-inquiry-head

National Audit Office (2013) 'Maternity services in England'. 8 November. URL: nao.org.uk/wp-content/uploads/2013/11/10259-001-Maternity-Services-Book-1.pdf

NHS Digital (2024) 'NHS Maternity Statistics, England, 2023–24'. 12 December. URL: digital.nhs.uk/data-and-information/publications/statistical/nhs-maternity-statistics/2023-24

O'Driscoll, K, Stringe, J M & Minogue, M (1973) 'Active management of labour'. *BMJ* 3(5872) 135–137. URL: pmc.ncbi.nlm.nih.gov/articles/PMC1586344/pdf/brmedj01567-0029.pdf

ONS (2025) 'Births in England and Wales: 2024'. URL: ons.gov.uk/peoplepopulationandcommunity/birthsdeathsandmarriages/livebirths/bulletins/birthsummarytablesenglandandwales/2024

Oxford Population Health (2024) 'Persistent inequalities remain in rates of stillbirth and neonatal deaths in the UK'. 15 July. URL: npeu.ox.ac.uk/news/2570-persistent-inequalities-remain-in-rates-of-stillbirth-and-neonatal-deaths-in-the-uk

Parliamentary and Health Care Service Ombudsman (2023) 'Repeated failings putting women and babies at risk'. 28 March. URL: www.ombudsman.org.uk/news-and-blog/news/repeated-failings-putting-women-and-babies-risk

Public Health England (2019) 'Health of women before and during pregnancy: Health behaviours, risk factors and inequalities' November. URL: assets.publishing.service.gov.uk/media/5dc00b22e5274a4a9a465013/Health_of_women_before_and_during_pregnancy_2019.pdf

RCOG (2015) 'The management of third and fourth degree perineal tears – Green-top Guideline No 29'. June. URL: rcog.org.uk/media/5jeb5hzu/gtg-29.pdf

RCOG (2016) 'Information for you: Birth options after previous caesarean section'. July. URL: rcog.org.uk/media/na3nigfb/pi-birth-options-after-previous-caesarean-section.pdf

RCOG (2018) 'Care of women with obesity in pregnancy – Green-top Guideline No 72'. November. URL: rcog.org.uk/guidance/browse-all-guidance/green-top-guidelines/care-of-women-with-obesity-in-pregnancy-green-top-guideline-no-72

Spendlove, Z (2017) 'Risk and boundary work in contemporary maternity care: Tensions and consequences'. *Health, Risk & Society* 20(1–2) 63–80. URL: doi.org/10.1080/13698575.2017.1398820

UK Government (2019) 'Perinatal mental health'. 25 October. URL: www.gov.uk/government/publications/better-mental-health-jsna-toolkit/4-perinatal-mental-health

Vousden, N, Bunch K et al (2024) 'Impact of maternal risk factors on ethnic disparities in maternal mortality: A national population-based cohort study'. *Lancet* 40 1–12. May. URL: pmc.ncbi.nlm.nih.gov/articles/PMC10998184/pdf/main.pdf

Zozzaro-Smith, P, Gray, L M et al (2014) 'Limitations of aneuploidy and anomaly detection in the obese patient'. *Journal of Clinical Medicine* 3 795–808. 17 July. URL: pmc.ncbi.nlm.nih.gov/articles/PMC4449658/pdf/jcm-03-00795.pdf

Chapter 7

Allen, A (2020) 'Whistleblower reveals maternity unit is still failing patients'. *Protect,* 24 August. URL: protect-advice.org.uk/whistleblower-reveals-maternity-unit-is-still-failing-patients

Bawa-Garba v General Medical Council (2018) URL: judiciary.uk/wp-content/uploads/2018/08/bawa-garba-v-gmc-final-judgment.pdf

BMA (2024a) 'Covid-19: The impact of the pandemic on the medical profession'. URL: bma.org.uk/media/2jhfvpgk/bma-covid-review-report-2-september-2024.pdf

BMA (2024b) 'Pay restoration for resident doctors in England'. URL: bma.org.uk/our-campaigns/resident-doctor-campaigns/pay-in-england/pay-restoration-for-resident-doctors-in-england

BMA (2025) 'BMA calls for creation of new medical register'. 23 June. URL: bma.org.uk/news-and-opinion/bma-calls-for-creation-of-new-medical-register

Council for Healthcare Regulatory Excellence (2012) 'Strategic review of Nursing and Midwifery Council'. 3 July. URL: nmc.org.uk/globalassets/sitedocuments/chre/120629-chre-final-report-for-nmc-strategic-review.pdf

Dyer, C (2021) 'GMC is accused of complacency about discrimination in its work'. *BMJ* 373. URL: bmj.com/content/373/bmj.n1595.full

Francis, R (2013) 'Report of the Mid Staffordshire NHS Foundation Trust Public Inquiry'. URL: assets.publishing.service.gov.uk/media/5a7c9bec40f0b65b3de09fde/0898_i.pdf

GMC (2022) 'GMC publishes report on deaths during investigations'. 3 March. URL: gmc-uk.org/news/news-archive/gmc-publishes-report-on-deaths-during-investigations

GMC (2024) 'Good medical practice'. URL: gmc-uk.org/-/media/documents/good-medical-practice-2024---english-102607294.pdf

Karim v General Medical Council (2021) 'Employment tribunals report'. URL: assets.publishing.service.gov.uk/media/6486b22fb32b9e000ca9653e/General_Medical_Council_v_Dr_O_M_A_Karim__2023__EAT_87.pdf

Lintern, S (2021a) 'Revealed: Women and babies at risk at hospital where doctors are censored and midwives fear working'. *The Independent,* 30 April URL: www.independent.co.uk/news/

health/maternity-safety-nhs-babies-worcester-b1835323.html

Lintern, S (2021b) 'Whistleblowers trigger downgrade of maternity unit over staff shortages'. *The Independent,* 19 February. URL: independent.co.uk/news/health/maternity-safety-nhs-staff-shortages-b1804016.html

Montgomery v Lanarkshire NHS Trust (2015) UK Supreme Court 15 March. URL: supremecourt.uk/uploads/uksc_2013_0136_judgment_fd5635b4cd.pdf

NHS England (2023) 'Working in partnership with people and communities: Statutory guidance'. May. URL: england.nhs.uk/long-read/working-in-partnership-with-people-and-communities-statutory-guidance

NHS England (2024) 'Feedback and complaints about NHS services'. URL: england.nhs.uk/contact-us/feedback-and-complaints/complaint

NHSR (2024) 'Annual reports and accounts 2023/4'. 31 March. URL: resolution.nhs.uk/wp-content/uploads/2024/07/NHS-Resolution-Annual-report-and-accounts_23-24_Access-1.pdf

Rimmer A (2023) 'One in three doctors experience suicidal thoughts during GMC investigation, survey finds'. *BMJ* 381:993. URL: bmj.com/content/381/bmj.p993

Talwar, D & Doherty, A (2025) 'Deaths of 56 babies at Leeds hospitals may have been preventable, BBC told.' BBC News, 17 January. URL: bbc.co.uk/news/articles/cq5gd48v10jo

The National Archives (1948) 'Difficulties between the Minister of Health and British Medical Association over the position of doctors etc in National Health Service'. URL: discovery.nationalarchives.gov.uk/details/r/C201118

Thomas, R (2021) 'Sandwell and West Birmingham NHS Trust – whistleblowers flag "toxic management" within maternity service'. *HSJ,* 10 March. URL: hsj.co.uk/sandwell-and-west-birmingham-hospitals-nhs-trust/

whistleblowers-flag-toxic-management-within-maternity-service/7029650.article

Thomas, R (2024) 'Scandal-hit nursing regulator accused of covering up critical internal review'. *The Independent,* 30 December. URL: independent.co.uk/news/health/nursing-midwifery-council-report-afzal-nhs-uk-b2666311.html

UK Parliament (2013) 'Written evidence from James Titcombe (CQC 05)'. URL: publications.parliament.uk/pa/cm201314/cmselect/cmhealth/526-i/526we06.htm

Woods, R (2022) 'Shrewsbury maternity scandal: "We've had to fight all the way for this"'. BBC News, 30 March. URL: bbc.co.uk/news/uk-england-shropshire-60926390

Chapter 8

Bick, D (2004) 'Caesarean section. Clinical guideline. National Collaborating Centre for Women's and Children's Health: commissioned by the National Institute for Clinical Excellence'. *Worldviews on Evidence-Based Nursing* 1(3) 198–9. URL: pubmed.ncbi.nlm.nih.gov/17163898

Campbell, D (2024) 'Poor NHS maternity care in danger of becoming "normalised", regulator warns'. *The Guardian*, 19 September. URL: theguardian.com/society/2024/sep/19/poor-nhs-maternity-care-in-danger-of-becoming-normalised-regulator-cqc

Church, E & Devereux, E (2024) 'Investigation: Massive increase in racial abuse against NHS staff'. *Nursing Times,* 10 June. URL: nursingtimes.net/workforce/investigation-massive-increase-in-racial-abuse-against-nhs-staff-10-06-2024

Department for International Development (2010) 'Fair society, healthy lives: Strategic review of health inequalities in England post-2010'. *The Marmot Review*, 1 January. URL: www.gov.uk/research-for-development-outputs/fair-society-healthy-lives-the-marmot-review-strategic-review-of-health-inequalities-in-england-post-2010

Iacobucci G (2022) 'Most black people in UK face discrimination from healthcare staff, survey finds'. *BMJ* 378:o2337. URL: bmj. com/content/378/bmj.o2337

Institute of Health Equity (2020) 'The Marmot Review 10 years on'. URL: instituteofhealthequity.org/resources-reports/ marmot-review-10-years-on/the-marmot-review-10-years-on-executive-summary.pdf

Jha, S & Power, E (eds) (2022) *Lessons from Medicolegal Cases in Obstetrics and Gynaecology: Improving clinical practice*. Cambridge University Press. URL: api.pageplace. de/preview/DT0400.9781108999403_A45557779/preview-9781108999403_A45557779.pdf

Johnson, J, Dunning, A et al (2020) 'Delivering unexpected news via obstetric ultrasound: A systematic review and meta-ethnographic synthesis of expectant parent and staff experiences'. URL: onlinelibrary.wiley.com/doi/epdf/10.1002/sono.12213

Kleine, R & Lewis, D (2019) 'The price of fear: Estimating the financial cost of bullying and harassment to the NHS in England'. *Public Money and Management* 39(3) 166–174. URL: tandfonline.com/doi/full/10.1080/09540962.2018.1535044

NCEPOD (2004) 'The 2004 report of the national confidential enquiry into patient outcome and death'. URL: ncepod.org. uk/2004report/Full_Report_2004.pdf

NHS England (2022) 'Combatting racial discrimination against minority ethnic nurses, midwives and nursing associates'. 6 December. URL: england.nhs.uk/long-read/ combatting-racial-discrimination-against-minority-ethnic-nurses-midwives-and-nursing-associates

NHS England (2023) 'New figures show NHS workforce most diverse it has ever been'. 22 February. URL: england.nhs.uk/2023/ 02/new-figures-show-nhs-workforce-most-diverse-it-has-ever-been

NHS England (2024) 'NHS execs more diverse than ever before'. 18 March. URL: england.nhs.uk/2024/03/nhs-execs-more-diverse-than-ever-before

NHS Race & Health Observatory (2022) 'Ethnic inequalities in healthcare: A rapid evidence review'. February. URL: nhsrho.org/wp-content/uploads/2023/05/RHO-Rapid-Review-Final-Report_.pdf

NHSR (2024a) 'Annual reports and accounts 2023/24'. 31 March. URL: resolution.nhs.uk/wp-content/uploads/2024/07/NHS-Resolution-Annual-report-and-accounts_23-24_Access-1.pdf

NHSR (2024b) 'NHS Resolution continues trend of resolving more cases without need for litigation'. 23 July. URL: resolution.nhs.uk/2024/07/23/nhs-resolution-continues-trend-of-resolving-more-cases-without-need-for-litigation

NHS Resolution (2025) 'Annual report and accounts 2024/25'. 17 July. URL: assets.publishing.service.gov.uk/media/6878fe277ea209168636391b/nhs-resolution-annual-report-and-accounts-2024-to-2025-hc1065.pdf

Pope, R (2018) 'Organizational silence in the NHS: "Hear no, see no, speak no"'. *Journal of Change Management* 19 1,45–66. URL: researchgate.net/publication/327445605_Organizational_Silence_in_the_NHS_'Hear_no_See_no_Speak_no'

RCM (2024) 'Midwives give 100,000 hours of free labour to the NHS per week to keep England's maternity services safe says RCM'. 11 June. URL: rcm.org.uk/media-releases/2024/06/midwives-give-100000-hours-of-free-labour-to-the-nhs-per-week-to-keep-englands-maternity-services-safe-says-rcm

RCOG (2021) 'Does bullying and undermining occur in O&G/maternity care?' URL: rcog.org.uk/careers-and-training/workforce/improving-workplace-behaviours/workplace-behaviour-toolkit/module-7-i-want-to-learn-more-about-workplace-behaviour/73-does-bullying-and-undermining-occur-inogmaternity-care

Rimmer, A (2015) 'Over 80% of doctors work unpaid overtime, NHS survey shows'. *BMJ* 350 1086. URL: bmj.com/content/350/bmj.h1086

Rimmer, A (2016) 'NHS must do more to tackle white male dominance of leadership roles, Labour Party says'. *BMJ* 354 i4610 URL: bmj.com/content/354/bmj.i4611

Ross, S, Jabbal, J et al (2020) 'Workforce race inequalities and inclusion in NHS providers'. The King's Fund, 7 July. URL: assets.kingsfund.org.uk/f/256914/x/eeb3fa7cd3/workforce_race_inequalities_inclusion_nhs_providers_2020.pdf

Stearn, E (2025) 'The 10 NHS Trusts you may think twice about giving birth in – as shocking report reveals areas with the most maternal injury complaints'. *Daily Mail*, 17 March. URL: web. archive.org/web/20250317155613/https://www.dailymail.co.uk/health/article-14506945/maternity-report-childbirth-injuries-dangerous-hospital-UK.html

The King's Fund (2015) 'Discrimination and NHS staff: Stepping bravely into the grey'. 16 December. URL: kingsfund.org.uk/insight-and-analysis/blogs/discrimination-nhs-staff-stepping-bravely-into-grey

Waters, A (2022) 'Racism is "at the root" of inequities in UK maternity care, finds inquiry'. *BMJ* 377 o1300. URL: bmj.com/content/377/bmj.o1300

Williams Report (2018) 'Gross negligence manslaughter in healthcare: The report of a rapid policy review'. June. URL: assets.publishing.service.gov.uk/government/uploads/system/uploads/attachment_data/file/717946/Williams_Report.pdf

Yau, C, Leigh, B et al (2020) 'Clinical negligence costs: Taking action to safeguard NHS sustainability'. *BMJ* 368:m552 URL: bmj.com/content/bmj/368/bmj.m552.full.pdf

Chapter 9

Betran, A P, Torloni, M R et al (2016) 'WHO statement on caesarean section rates'. *BJOG* 123 667–670. URL: obgyn.onlinelibrary.wiley.com/doi/10.1111/1471-0528.13526

Bliss (2024) 'Full term babies needing neonatal care'. URL: bliss.org.uk/research-campaigns/neonatal-care-statistics/statistics-for-babies-admitted-to-neonatal-units-at-full-term

Crossan, K A, Geraghty, S & Balding, K (2023) 'The use of gender-neutral language in maternity settings: A narrative literature review'. *British Journal of Midwifery* 31(9). URL: britishjournalofmidwifery.com/content/literature-review/the-use-of-gender-neutral-language-in-maternity-settings-a-narrative-literature-review

Dahlen, H G, Drandic, D et al (2022) 'Supporting midwifery is the answer to the wicked problems in maternity care'. *Lancet* 10 951–952. URL: thelancet.com/action/showPdf?pii=S2214-109X%2822%2900183-8

Freemantle, N, Ray, D et al (2015) 'Increased mortality associated with weekend hospital admission: A case for expanded seven day services?' *BMJ* 2015 351. URL: bmj.com/content/351/bmj.h4596.full

Gilbert, P (2025) 'Compassion fatigue in NHS or burnout?'. *The Guardian,* 5 January. URL: theguardian.com/society/2025/jan/05/compassion-fatigue-in-the-nhs-or-burnout

Goto, E (2020) 'Symphysis-fundal height to identify large-for-gestational-age and macrosomia: A meta-analysis'. *Journal of Obstetrics and Gynaecology* 40(7) 929–935. URL: pubmed.ncbi.nlm.nih.gov/31814480

Group B Strep Support (2025) 'Group B Strep infection in babies'. URL: gbss.org.uk/info-support/group-b-strep-infection/after-gbs-infection

Jain, M, Chkipov, P et al (2022) 'Online Patient Information for Hysterectomies: A Systematic Environmental Scan of Quality and Readability'. *Journal of Obstetrics and Gynaecology Canada* 44(8):870–876. URL: jogc.com/article/S1701-2163(22)00331-0

Lampert A, Wien, K et al (2016) 'Guidance on how to achieve comprehensible patient information leaflets in four steps'. *Journal of the International Society for Quality in Health Care* 28(5) 634–638. URL: europepmc.org/article/MED/27512127

NHS England (2023) 'Changes to cancer waiting times standards from 1 October 2023'. 17 August. URL: england.nhs.uk/

wp-content/uploads/2023/08/PRN00654ii-changes-to-cancer-waiting-times-standards-from-1-october-2023-letter.pdf

NHS England (2024) 'Patient safety incident response framework and supporting guidance'. 25 July. URL: england.nhs.uk/publication/patient-safety-incident-response-framework-and-supporting-guidance

NHS Inform (2025) 'How to look after your pelvic floor'. URL: nhsinform.scot/ready-steady-baby/pregnancy/looking-after-yourself-and-your-baby/how-to-look-after-your-pelvic-floor

NHS Patient Information (2025) 'Chestfeeding if you're trans or non-binary'. URL: nhs.uk/pregnancy/having-a-baby-if-you-are-lgbt-plus/chestfeeding-if-youre-trans-or-non-binary/

Parket, C (2022) 'Maternity scandal: Bosses at disgraced Shrewsbury NHS Trust went on to lucrative health jobs'. *Times*, 30 March. URL: thetimes.com/uk/healthcare/article/bosses-at-disgraced-shrewsbury-nhs-trust-went-on-to-lucrative-health-jobs-zr35g5f2j

Pezaro, S, Pendleton, J et al (2023) 'Gender-inclusive language in midwifery and perinatal services: A guide and argument for justice'. *Birth*. URL: pubmed.ncbi.nlm.nih.gov/38822631

Pietrzykowski, T & Smilowska, K (2021) 'The reality of informed consent: Empirical studies on patient comprehension-systematic review'. *Trials* 14:22(1) 57. URL: pubmed.ncbi.nlm.nih.gov/33446265

RCM (2021) 'Making maternity services safer: Nurturing a positive culture'. September. URL: rcm.org.uk/wp-content/uploads/2024/06/solution_series_4_making_maternity_sevices_safer_nurturing_a_positive_culture_.pdf

RCM (2025) 'Government announces pay award for RCM members in England, Wales and Northern Ireland'. 23 May. URL: rcm.org.uk/media-releases/2025/05/government-announces-pay-award-for-rcm-members-in-england-wales-and-northern-ireland

RCOG (2023) 'Good practice paper on maternity triage'. 11 December. URL: rcog.org.uk/news/rcog-publishes-good-practice-paper-on-maternity-triage

Robert, P J, Ho J J et al (2015) 'Symphysial fundal height (SFH) measurement in pregnancy for detecting abnormal fetal growth'. *Cochrane Database Syst Rev*(9): CD008136. URL: pmc.ncbi. nlm.nih.gov/articles/PMC6465049/pdf/CD008136.pdf

Silverman, J & Kinnersley, P (2010) 'Doctors' non-verbal behaviour in consultations: Look at the patient before you look at the computer'. *British Journal of General Practice* 60(571) 76–78. URL: pubmed.ncbi.nlm.nih.gov/20132698

Tam N T, Huy N T et al (2015) 'Participants' understanding of informed consent in clinical trials over three decades: Systematic review and meta-analysis'. *Bulletin of the World Health Organization* 1:93(3) 186–98H. URL: pubmed.ncbi.nlm.nih. gov/25883410

UK Government (2024) 'Screening for Down's syndrome, Edwards' syndrome and Patau's syndrome'. 16 December. URL: www.gov.uk/government/publications/ fetal-anomaly-screening-programme-handbook/screening-for-downs-syndrome-edwards-syndrome-and-pataus-syndrome--3

Urbankova, I, Grohregin, K et al (2019) 'The effect of the first vaginal birth on pelvic floor anatomy and dysfunction'. *International Urogynecology Journal* 30(10) 1689–1696. URL: pmc.ncbi.nlm.nih.gov/articles/PMC6795623

Chapter 10

Anderson, M, O'Neill, C et al (2021) 'Securing a sustainable and fit-for-purpose UK health and care workforce'. *Lancet* 397(10288) 1992–2011. URL: pubmed.ncbi.nlm.nih. gov/33965066

Barker, S (2025) 'UK private medical insurance sign-ups near-record high amid NHS backlog'. *City AM,* 7 February. URL: cityam. com/uk-private-medical-insurance-sign-ups-near-record-high-amid-nhs-backlog

BBC (2018) 'The NHS at 70: A timeline in pictures'. 5 July. URL: bbc.co.uk/news/in-pictures-44613043

BBC News (2020) 'Coronavirus: Boris Johnson "owes his life to NHS staff"'. 12 April. URL: bbc.co.uk/news/uk-52258980

Bielecki, A, & Nieszporska, S (2019) 'Analysis of healthcare systems by using systemic approach'. *Complexity* article ID 6807140. URL: onlinelibrary.wiley.com/doi/epdf/10.1155/2019/6807140

Bootle, R, Ramanauskas, B & Sweetman, B (2025) 'The NHS – a Suitable Case for Treatment? The fifth part of Policy Exchange's Policy Programme for Prosperity'. July. URL: policyexchange. org.uk/wp-content/uploads/The.NHS_.A.Suitable.Case_.For_. Treatment.pdf

Bramwell, K (2023) 'Ambulance service being misused, paramedics say'. BBC News, 11 January. URL: bbc.co.uk/news/health-64136691

Butler, P (2020) 'A million volunteer to help NHS and others during Covid-19 outbreak'. *The Guardian,* 13 April. URL: theguardian. com/society/2020/apr/13/a-million-volunteer-to-help-nhs-and-others-during-covid-19-lockdown

Clarke, R (2024) 'Wes Streeting, you must have a better plan for ailing hospitals than public humiliation'. *The Guardian,* 13 November. URL: theguardian.com/commentisfree/2024/nov/13/ wes-streeting-hospitals-league-tables-nhs-staff

Commission on the future of the NHS (2021) 'Re-laying the foundations for an equitable and efficient health and care service after Covid-19'. *Lancet,* 6 May. URL: thelancet.com/ commissions/future-NHS

DHSC (2020) 'Busting bureaucracy: Empowering frontline staff by reducing excess bureaucracy in the health and care system in England'. 24 November. URL: www.gov.uk/ government/calls-for-evidence/reducing-bureaucracy-in-the-health-and-social-care-system-call-for-evidence/outcome/ busting-bureaucracy-empowering-frontline-staff-by-reducing-excess-bureaucracy-in-the-health-and-care-system-in-england

Gregory, A (2022) 'Millions of UK patients forced to go private amid record NHS waiting lists'. *The Guardian,* 11 September.

URL: theguardian.com/society/2022/sep/11/millions-uk-patients-forced-private-nhs-waiting-lists

Jones, R (2020) 'UK volunteering soars during coronavirus crisis'. *The Guardian*, 25 May. URL: theguardian.com/society/2020/may/26/uk-volunteering-coronavirus-crisis-community-lockdown

Knox, T (2022) 'International Health Care Outcomes Index 2022'. URL: civitas.org.uk/content/files/International-Health-Care-Outcomes-Index-FINAL.pdf

Lintern, S (2024) 'NHS told to cut spending on doctors and nurses to save £4.5bn'. *The Sunday Times*, 31 March. URL: thetimes.com/uk/article/nhs-told-to-cut-spending-on-doctors-and-nurses-to-save-45bn-sbgk7k02d

NHS Digital (2024) 'Data on written complaints in the NHS 2023–24'. 17 October. URL: digital.nhs.uk/data-and-information/publications/statistical/data-on-written-complaints-in-the-nhs/2023-24

NHS England (2019) 'Missed GP appointments costing NHS millions'. 2 January. URL: england.nhs.uk/2019/01/missed-gp-appointments-costing-nhs-millions

NHS England (2022) 'NHS announces £127 million maternity boost for patients and families'. 24 March. URL: england.nhs.uk/2022/03/nhs-announces-127m-maternity-boost-for-patients-and-families

NHS England (2023) 'England's NHS mental health services treat record 3.8 million people last year'. 10 October. URL: england.nhs.uk/2024/10/englands-nhs-mental-health-services-treat-record-3-8-million-people-last-year

NHS England (2024) 'Where to get urgent help for mental health'. URL: nhs.uk/nhs-services/mental-health-services/where-to-get-urgent-help-for-mental-health/

OECD (2023) 'Health at a glance'. URL: oecd.org/en/publications/health-at-a-glance-2023_7a7afb35-en/full-report/mortality-following-ischaemic-stroke_31210125.html

ONS (2023a) 'Visits to and from the UK for the purpose
of medical treatment, 2021'. URL: ons.gov.uk/
peoplepopulationandcommunity/leisureandtourism/adhocs/
1019visitstoandfromukforthepurposeofmedicaltreatment2021

ONS (2023b) 'Rising ill-health and economic inactivity because of
long-term sickness, UK: 2019 to 2023'. 26 July. URL: ons.gov.uk/
releases/risingillhealthandeconomicinactivityduetolongtermsick
nessuk2019to2023

ONS (2024) 'Accident and emergency wait times across the UK:
2024'. 28 February. URL: ons.gov.uk/peoplepopulationand

communityhealthandsocialcare/healthcaresystem/articles/
accidentandemergencywaittimesacrosstheuk/2024-02-28

Papanicolas, I, Mossialos, E et al (2019) 'Performance of UK
National Health Service compared with other high income
countries: Observational study'. *BMJ* 367 l6326. URL: pubmed.
ncbi.nlm.nih.gov/31776110

Pickles, K (2024) 'Health Secretary Victoria Atkins reveals "dark
corners" of NHS left her "worried and frightened" during
pregnancy'. *Daily Mail,* 17 January. URL: dailymail.co.uk/health/
article-12974527/Health-Secretary-Victoria-Atkins-reveals-dark-
corners-NHS-left-worried-frightened-pregnancy

Power, J, Phillips, S & Carroll, S (2022) 'Just about managing:
The role of effective management and leadership in improving
NHS performance and productivity'. *Policy Exchange.* URL:
policyexchange.org.uk/wp-content/uploads/Just-About-
Managing-2.pdf

Rose Report (2015) 'NHS Leadership Review – better leadership
for tomorrow'. June. URL: assets.publishing.service.gov.
uk/government/uploads/system/uploads/attachment_data/
file/445738/Lord_Rose_NHS_Report_acc.pdf

Royal College of Emergency Medicine (2024) 'Almost 300 deaths
a week in 2023 associated with long A&E waits despite
UEC Recovery Plan'. 1 April. URL: rcem.ac.uk/press-release/

almost-300-deaths-a-week-in-2023-associated-with-long-ae-waits-despite-uecrecovery-plan

Sommerlad, N (2024) 'Crisis-hit NHS spent "unacceptable" £140m on management consultants in four years'. *The Mirror*, 9 December. URL: mirror.co.uk/news/uk-news/crisis-hit-nhs-spent-unacceptable-34279525

Tanne, J H (2023) 'Nearly six million women in the US live in maternity care deserts' *BMJ* 382 1878. URL: pubmed.ncbi.nlm.nih.gov/37580083

The Health Foundation (2021) 'Why our perceptions of the NHS matter'. 1 April. URL: health.org.uk/features-and-opinion/blogs/why-our-perceptions-of-the-nhs-matter

The King's Fund (2024a) 'Waiting times for elective (non-urgent) treatment: Referral to treatment (RTT)'. URL: kingsfund.org.uk/insight-and-analysis/data-and-charts/waiting-times-non-urgent-treatment

The King's Fund (2024b) 'Public satisfaction with the NHS and social care in 2023'. URL: kingsfund.org.uk/insight-and-analysis/reports/public-satisfaction-nhs-social-care-2023

Triggle, N (2014) 'One-fifth of patients "admit to misusing A&E units"'. BBC News, 4 March. URL: bbc.co.uk/news/health-26425453

UK Parliament (2024) 'Women and Equalities Committee: Women's reproductive health conditions'. House of Commons – First Report of Session 2024–25. URL: committees.parliament.uk/publications/45909/documents/228040/default

EU Safety Representative: euComply OÜ Pärnu mnt 139b-14 11317 Tallinn
Estonia hello@eucompliancepartner.com +33 756 90241

www.ingramcontent.com/pod-product-compliance
Lightning Source LLC
Chambersburg PA
CBHW041733200326
41518CB00020B/2585